Doctor in your Pocket

A Handbook of the Human Body

ANATOMY
(HOW IS IT BUILT?)
PHYSIOLOGY AND BIOCHEMISTRY
(HOW DOES IT WORK?)
PATHOLOGY
(WHAT CAN GO WRONG WITH IT?)
WHEN TO CALL THE DOCTOR
WHAT TO SAY
"DOCTOR SPEAK" VOCABULARY
SHARE IN YOUR CARE

Ralph R. Gold, M.D.

ISBN : 1-4392-3102-8
ISBN-13: 9781439231029

To order additional copies, please contact us.
BookSurge
www.booksurge.com
1-866-308-6235
orders@booksurge.com

TABLE OF CONTENTS

ACKNOWLEDGMENTS

This book has been a labor of love from its inception, which was almost immediately upon my retirement in 2001. The incentive to write was the awareness of my very good fortune in having had such a rich and varied career as a Family Physician for so many wonderful patients, and a teacher on the clinical faculty of the U.C.L.A. School Of Medicine. The greatest satisfaction from all those encounters was the memory of having communicated successfully with so many people in varied walks of life. For this I will be eternally grateful to my patients and to the medical students and Family Practice residents whom I was privileged to teach. I am firmly convinced that the ability to communicate with patients and their families is the greatest asset that any physician can have and is, in fact, a basic requirement for a successful career in medicine.

To write a book encompassing so many aspects of the body was a daunting task. I am extremely grateful to John K. Cherry, M.D., my medical school classmate at the University Of Southern California and a highly respected surgeon at Scripps Hospital in La Jolla, California for his invaluable consultation in keeping the anatomic and physiologic descriptions accurate.

The rigors of having a book published for one with failing eyesight, such as myself, were greatly lessened by the generous help given by Mr. John Delaney, owner of OVAC, a facility dealing with instruments of great assistance to the visually impaired, in Cathedral City, California.

I am fortunate to have the love and support of my five daughters. For above-and-beyond assistance in conquering the challenges of word processing, I am grateful to my daughter Pamela Gold Bothwell. And for her unstinting help throughout the production of this book, I am grateful to my daughter Meredith Gold.

The one individual who should get special recognition for assistance in the writing of this book is my wife, Heather, who has put up with the years of my agonizing over its creation. Without her patience, encouragement and advice it could not have been written.

INTRODUCTION

How does the heart really work? What does "heart attack" really mean? What is a stroke? Just what is it and what does it do? How do the lungs work? What is a ruptured disc? How does a pregnancy develop in the body? How do birth control pills work? What is leukemia? How do the eyes and the ears really work? The answers to those and many more questions are in this book.

Those are the kinds of questions that a family doctor hears every day. They are good questions, and are entitled to good answers. There we find a problem. In the present era of "managed" medical care few doctors have the time to even listen carefully to questions or to give complete and satisfactory answers and advice.

That is the chief motivating factor that led to the writing of this book. A well-informed and intelligent patient has a better chance of staying healthy and happy than one who carries fears and anxieties about his or her body because of the lack of good information. The book was also written for the benefit of those highly motivated people who work in medically related fields such as paramedics, technicians and nurses. Those individuals often have a great deal of responsibility but lack sufficient information about the body or the disease process to be confident and effective in their work.

This book is designed as a handbook for those who need to know and perhaps more importantly, for those who simply want to know more about the body. There is description of the anatomy of each part and each system of the body (how it is built), its physiology and biochemistry (how it works) and the pathology (the most common diseases and disorders) of each organ and system. That information is organized into chapters for each system of the body, making it integrated and easily accessed. The information is given in a compact form that is readily understandable. The technical details are extensive. The correct medical terminology, "Doctor Speak", is used throughout and translated into plain English.

It is my hope that the greatest contribution of this book will be to give the readers enough knowledge of the body and enough technical language to be better able to communicate with the doctor, and in that way to better take charge of their own lives.

HOW TO BEST READ AND USE THIS BOOK

Each chapter will be devoted to a different system of the body. First will be a discussion of the anatomy of that system. Wherever applicable that will be accompanied by a discussion of the physiology and biochemistry of that system. That will describe how the system is built and how it works. Following that there will be a presentation of the most common disorders that involve each system, referred to as the pathology of that system.

There will be no specific recommendation for treatment of the disorders, other than suggestions for nonprescription medications to treat early symptoms. The word "symptoms" in correct medical terms refers to those effects or complaints noted by the patient, such as pain or weakness. Those things which can be noted externally by an observer, such as fever, swelling, or tenderness when the affected part is touched or pressed are called signs. Quite often the reader will be advised of when to call for professional help and what vocabulary to use.

As a general rule I will first use the common name for any part of the anatomy or any medical condition. That will be accompanied by the proper name in medical terminology (Doctor Speak). That name will be enclosed in parentheses. This will help the reader to build a vocabulary of medical terms.

INFLAMMATION (A BASIC CONCEPT)

Before we begin our study of all the systems of the body it's important to understand the process of inflammation. That word is familiar to most people, but really understood by very few. It will reappear frequently in this book, so let's go through a simple explanation of how inflammation works.

Inflammation is the body's first line of defense against most injuries, whether due to injury or illness, in any part of the body. It's easy to see in the redness of a sore throat, or in the swelling of a sprained ankle or knee. It is most easily seen in the blistering of a hand after work with a shovel, but very difficult to appreciate in the case of acute appendicitis or a stroke that damages the brain. As widely different as those injuries are, the process of inflammation is basically the same. The events in the process of inflammation are as follows:

1. Injury of body tissue can occur from any source, such as thermal or chemical burns, viral or bacterial infection, sprains or fractures, or blood clot in a vein or artery. All of those injuries cause the affected

tissues to release a chemical compound called histamine, or a "Histamine-like substance."

2. The presence of that substance causes local capillaries, which are tiny blood vessels to dilate. The capillary dilation stretches the spaces between the cells that form the walls of the capillaries, allowing blood plasma to flow out of the capillaries. That fluid provides cushioning of the surrounding tissue. The most easily seen examples of that are "water on the knee" after a sprain, or the similar swelling of an injured ankle, or a blister from friction on a hand.
3. Blood plasma contains protective protein molecules called "antibodies" that are released into the site of injury. As the capillaries continue to dilate they allow passage of blood cells into the site of injury. Those will fight infecting organisms, if any. As the result of this process there is often local redness, swelling, heat, and pain in the site of the injury.

As we progress through the systems of the body you will encounter reference to inflammation quite frequently. These basic events apply to the inflammatory process in any part of the body.

TERMINOLOGY COMMONLY USED THROUGHOUT THIS BOOK

The word "cancer" is familiar to everyone. It will be used many times in this book. There is a way to describe different forms of cancer that has evolved over many years. In a very brief form this is it. Based on Greek roots, the suffix "oma" means swelling, or lump of any sort. The Greek prefix "carcin" means cancer, in any usage. The word "CARCINOMA" is the full Greek word for cancer. Depending on the tissue of origin other prefixes are added. The word "ADENOCARCINOMA" means cancer of glandular origin. This is one of the most common forms of cancer and the word is used a lot. Thus "HEMATOMA" refers to a swelling due to a collection of blood. It can be a "blood blister" on a hand or a huge swelling inside, due to major internal bleeding. The word "MALIGNANT" always refers to a growth that is cancerous, whereas the word "BENIGN" refers to a growth that is not cancerous, and also to a condition which will have a favorable outcome.

This explanation will be of help as you go through the book. You will see that "carcinoma" is a condition that can occur to virtually every part of the body, and will be preceded of followed by the name of the tissue of origin, such as "gastric carcinoma", (stomach) or "pulmonary carcinoma" (lung). It gets easier to understand as you go on.

The suffix meaning inflammation is "itis." This applies to inflammation anywhere in the body. Thus, inflammation of the throat is "pharyngitis", of the nose "rhinitis", of the bronchial passages, "bronchitis", and of the appendix "appendicitis." This will be consistent throughout the book, regardless of whether the inflammation is due to an allergic reaction, an infection, or a physical injury, such as bursitis.

The language of medicine and the medically related sciences is filled with terminology. Some of the terms are modern, and some have persisted from medical antiquity. Some of the words act as a form of shorthand in which an entire idea or concept is compressed into a single word. Physicians commonly use this form of shorthand. Many physicians use words that are not understood by their patients and the families of their patients.

This book will contain proper terminology that is specific and descriptive throughout, with the translation into common English whenever possible.

Chapter One
THE RESPIRATORY SYSTEM

This system consists of those parts of the body that function in the taking in of air and the transferring of oxygen to the tissues of the body, then the transfer of carbon dioxide and other spent gases from the body and their exhaustion through the lungs.

The respiratory system is the first to be discussed because there is no part of the body that is more frequently in need of medical care. The problems begin at birth with congenital defects and malformations. Then, often seen in infancy, are respiratory infections. The problems get more complicated in childhood with tonsillitis, croup, ear infections, asthma and bronchitis, and they continue throughout life with pneumonia, pleurisy, emphysema, and cancer.

None of those are rare disorders, and most need medical attention. The reader will most likely find information that will be of personal use, as well as good basic information, and explanations of conditions that you have heard about for many years past.

The route that we will take in our tour is to follow the pathway taken by air in and out of the respiratory system. That begins with the upper airway, including the mouth and nasal passages and throat, then goes on to the nasopharynx (the place where the nose and throat come together), including the passages to the sinuses and ears. Next we come to the larynx and vocal cords. Then we will discuss the lower airway which includes the trachea, the bronchi and bronchioles and finally the air sacs (alveoli). Air containing spent gases is exhausted via the reverse route.

ANATOMY AND PHYSIOLOGY OF THE RESPIRATORY SYSTEM

The passage of air through the mouth is fairly straightforward. Air enters through the mouth and passes into the throat (Pharynx). The lining of the entire airway, with the exception of the mouth, is a mucous membrane, which is a thin, smooth, shiny sheet of tissue that is densely filled with mucus glands. Those glands produce thin fluid called mucus. That fluid, though it appears to be watery, is far from being pure water. It contains protein and carbohydrate substances that moisten the air and protect the airway from injury by noxious substances and potential invaders, such as virus, bacteria, and fungus organisms.

The passage of air through the nose is different. The nasal airway on the sides away from midline (lateral sides) bears a series of ridges, called turbinates which greatly increase the surface area of the nasal airway. The exposure of the incoming air to that added area of mucous membrane moistens the air significantly. The inner, (medial) side of the nasal airway is a mucous membrane that lies against the thick tissue of the nasal septum that divides the two sides of the nose. The septum is made of cartilage, which is moderately flexible. At the rear the septum connects with the nasal bones that are rigid, and more susceptible to injury.

The nasal airway does much more to moisten the incoming air and to expose it to the protective mucus than does the oral airway. As a general rule, it is better to breathe through the nose than through the mouth while at rest. During heavy exertion it becomes necessary to breathe through the mouth because that pathway offers less resistance to deep and rapid breathing.

The place where the nasal and oral airways come together is called the nasopharynx. That area is very complicated anatomically because it is the meeting place of the passages leading to the sinuses and the Eustachean tubes that lead to the middle ear.

There are eight sinuses, four on each side of the head. They are hollow cavities, lined with mucous membranes. There is no specific known function of the sinuses, other than to increase the resonance of the voice, but they are frequent sources of infection and allergic swelling. The maxillary sinuses are located just below the eye sockets, (orbits). The frontal sinuses lie just above the orbits. The ethmoid and sphenoid sinuses are deeper in the skull, behind the orbits. They all drain through small passages into the nasopharynx.

The Eustachean tubes are small passages that begin at the nasopharynx and travel through the bone of the skull, ending within the middle ear. The middle ear is a closed box between the external ear and the inner ear. Those structures will be discussed in detail in the chapter of the organs of special senses. As the flow of air continues through the respiratory tract it passes through the pharynx (the back of the throat), through a structure called the epiglottis, and into the larynx.

The epiglottis is a strong fibro-muscular cap, supplied with sensory nerves that can sense the presence of any solid or liquid matter in the passageway to the lungs. If that is the case, a healthy epiglottis shuts down the airway to the lungs, causing violent coughing to expel that matter, thus protecting the lungs from serious damage.

Another important function of the epiglottis is that it participates with the adjacent strong muscles in holding the opening from the trachea closed. That is necessary in order to build up pressure within the lungs, then to release that pressure abruptly. That enables us to cough in order to clear the airway.

At times it is also necessary to hold and increase the pressure within the lungs, as in straining at a bowel movement. That is done by closing the epiglottis and straining to push downward. (That, in Doctor Speak, is called the Valsalva maneuver). The result is that the diaphragm is pushed downward, increasing the pressure within the abdominal cavity, helping to empty stool from the bowel.

Located just below the epiglottis is the larynx, home of the vocal cords. Those are flexible ligaments, held within the cartilage of the larynx by muscle tissue. The vocal cords can tighten or loosen upon commands from the brain. They vibrate when air is forced through them from the lungs and trachea, producing sound. The size of the vocal cords and tension placed upon them by their attached muscles are responsible for the sound of the voice and the wonderful ability to produce music found in some people.

The trachea is a semi-rigid tube that extends from the larynx toward the lungs. Its state of rigidity is maintained by rings of cartilage that can be felt by your fingers on the front of your neck. The trachea divides into right and left branches which connect with the bronchial passages. It is lined with a mucous membrane, and is a very wide passage. In the average adult the trachea is often in excess of an inch in diameter and of course, is much narrower in infants and children. The function of the trachea is to conduct air in and out of the lungs.

THE LUNGS

All of the discussion to this point has described the upper airway. Beginning with the lower end of the trachea we enter the area of the lungs. That consists of the lower trachea, the bronchi, the bronchioles, and the alveoli. The membranous structures of the chest are essential in the mechanics of breathing and will also be discussed here.

The trachea divides into right and left branches, becoming progressively smaller in caliber, but still supplied with cartilaginous rings. At their distal ends the right and left branches make connection with the bronchi. The bronchial passages begin at the trachea, and extend deep into the lungs on both sides. The diameter of those passages becomes smaller as they pass deeper into the lungs. At their largest diameter they are called bronchi. As they become smaller they are called bronchioles.

The bronchial passages all have a muscular outer wall and a lining of mucous membrane. The muscle walls enable those passages to go into spasm, reducing the caliber of the airway. The narrowing of the passageway serves to prevent particles that may have entered the airway from penetrating deeper, in that way protecting the alveolar air sacs. The ability to go into spasm becomes very important in conditions such as asthma.

The smallest bronchioles make connections with the final structures in the depth of the lungs, the alveoli, which are the terminal air sacs.

The alveolus, (singular) is the place where the real business of breathing is conducted. The alveoli are gossamer sacs of nearly transparent tissue. There are millions of alveoli in each lung. Each alveolus is supplied with a tiny blood vessel called a capillary. The walls of those blood vessels are so thin that gases pass through them into the thin- walled alveoli.

Blood returning from every part of the body is rich in carbon dioxide and other waste gases. Those gases flow out of the capillaries and through their thin walls into the alveoli. With every exhalation (expiration) those waste gases pass into the bronchioles, then into the bronchi, then into the trachea to be exhausted into the upper airway, the pharynx, and out of the body via the nose and mouth.

Immediately afterward, in the inhalation, (inspiration) phase of breathing, oxygen-rich air enters the blood from the alveoli by the reverse of the above process. Oxygen is transferred from the alveoli into the capillaries. Within the capillaries are red blood cells, loaded with an iron pigment called heme. Heme pigment in the red blood cells accepts oxygen from the alveoli. Freshly oxygenated blood has a bright red color. Venous blood, poor in oxygen and rich in carbon dioxide has a bluish-red appearance. From the capillaries the red blood cells flow into the arterioles, then into the arteries. The arteries carry the blood throughout the body where it releases the oxygen to all the bodily tissues via the arterioles and the capillaries. At that point the heme pigment in the red blood cells accepts waste gases, chiefly carbon dioxide from the tissues to be carried back to the lungs via the venous system.

This process occurs twenty-four hours of every day, from fifteen to twenty times every minute. The exchange of gases within the red blood cells is enabled by the presence of an enzyme called carbonic anhydrase. The chemical reactions involved are very complicated, yet are completed in milliseconds.

Throughout this book you will encounter many examples of very complicated events, including chemical reactions, electrical switching and routing, and some sub-intellectual brain functions that are unbelievably complex, yet occur in milliseconds of time. The real complexity of the body is truly awe-inspiring.

The tour of the respiratory system has thus far been confined to those passages which conduct air in and out of the body. There are other structures that are indispensable to the process of breathing, and can be affected by disease states. We will look at a few.

The intercostal muscles located between the ribs are responsible for the flaring out of the ribs to increase the capacity of the lungs during inspiration, when they contract. When those muscles relax the chest size becomes smaller, emptying the lungs.

The diaphragm is a broad sheet of thick muscle which separates the chest cavity from the abdominal cavity. When the diaphragm is contracted it moves in a downward direction, expanding the size of the chest cavity during inspiration. During expiration the diaphragm relaxes in an upward (superior) direction's reducing the capacity of the chest cavity, and pushing out the spent air.

The pleura are a thin smooth serous membrane. It is called "serous" because of its smooth and slippery quality. The pleural membrane lines the inside of the chest cavity within the ribs. It extends to the lungs, which it envelops with its smooth slippery membrane. The presence of that serous membrane allows the lungs to slide within the chest cavity as they expand with the incoming air and contract during expiration.

We have finished our anatomical and physiological tour of the most important parts of the respiratory system. Of course there are many more parts, especially the nerves that control breathing, but the structures described here are the most important ones to know at this point. They all can be involved in various disease states, which we will discuss next.

DISORDERS OF THE RESPIRATORY SYSTEM

"It woke us in the middle of the night, a sound coming from the room of our three year-old daughter. She had appeared to be healthy and happy earlier when we kissed her goodnight. Her breathing was very fast and strained, with a high-pitched squeak and whistle sound. She was crying and fighting for breath. My husband picked her up and took her into the shower with hot water making a lot of steam while I called 911 for help. The paramedics got there fast and gave her shots and oxygen that helped her breathing. They rushed her to Children's Hospital where they gave her intensive treatment. Her breathing quieted down and she fell asleep. We were able to take her home the next day with a lot of medicine. The diagnosis was croup, which they called acute tracheobronchitis."

In the course of a day in a family physician's office one can see babies and young children who inhale things and put things up their noses and in their ears. They get croup and kindergarten colds and "strep throats." Older people have bronchitis, asthma, pneumonia and sinusitis. Senior citizens get pneumonia, pleurisy, emphysema and, tragically, cancer. Actually, most people are susceptible to most of the above and lots more. Let's look at the parts of this system of the body that are most likely to have the most common problems.

We will follow the same pathway as in the previous section on anatomy and physiology, beginning with the lips and nares. The most commonly encountered, and the most serious disorders will be discussed.

The Mouth and Nasopharynx

The lips and mouth do not have any serious disorders that affect respiration. The chief problem involving them is virus infection, the most common of which is Herpes Simplex. This infection appears as "cold sores" on the lips, and ulcers of the lining membrane of the mouth. These are painful, but not considered a serious threat to health. There are prescription medications and nonprescription remedies that are helpful. For very severely painful sores it's best that you contact your doctor for an antiviral prescription medication that is usually quite effective. "Cold sores" on the lips tend to recur, especially after severe sun exposure. The best explanation for that is the tendency of the virus that causes the infection to remain dormant in the deeper layers of the lips, and to be activated by sun exposure.

There are two main types of conditions that affect the passages of the nose. They are allergy and infection. First let's talk about allergy.

There is a discussion of allergy and the science of immunology in a later chapter of this book. Allergic reactions are extremely common in the respiratory system. The most common signs and symptoms are usually swelling of the mucous membranes, causing obstruction of the airway, that we call stuffy nose, profuse secretion of nasal mucus, that we call runny nose, and obstruction of the openings of the sinuses and Eustachean tubes in the nasopharynx. The latter can lead to sinusitis and ear infections.

The term "infection" is very specific. It refers to the invasion of the body by a living, infectious organism. In order of frequency those organisms are viruses, bacteria, and fungi.

In the nose the most common infecting organisms are viruses, such as the common cold virus. Bacterial organisms are less frequently involved in nasal infections and fungus organisms are rarely involved. In virus infections the antigen-antibody reaction often occurs, because viruses are very small protein molecules that the body's immune defenses can combat effectively in most cases. (See chapter 12)

Bacterial infections of the nasal airway resemble viral infections, but are much less common. The body defends against them by means of the antibody reaction, and also by the release of certain cells from the blood stream that attack and destroy bacteria. To supplement the body's own defenses against bacterial infection there is a wide array of antibiotics.

At this point I would like to enter a plea against the over-use of antibiotics in respiratory infections. Most infections of the nose and throat are caused by viruses which are totally resistant to any antibiotic. In most cases the body's own defenses will overcome viral respiratory infections. In a small percentage of cases the infection is due to a bacterial organism. It's common sense to avoid using a powerful drug for a futile treatment. It's best, in most cases, to have a culture taken of the nose or throat to confirm the presence of a bacterial organism prior to taking an antibiotic. This greatly reduces the likelihood of creating allergy to the antibiotic in case of future need for that antibiotic. It also is very important to avoid the exposure of "innocent bacteria" that live normally in the respiratory tract, and that are not involved in the infection to antibiotics which could cause them to acquire a resistance against the antibiotic in case of future infection.

The space behind the mouth is the throat, (pharynx). Any inflammation of the pharynx is called "pharyngitis", true to our nomenclature of inflammation. Inflammations of the throat in most cases are due to infection. Viral organisms are the most common cause of pharyngitis, although there is a significant incidence of bacterial infection. This requires antibiotic treatment after proper identification.

In the very back of the pharynx on either side lie structures called the pharyngeal tonsils and adenoids. They are essentially lymph nodes, a visible portion of the lymphatic system. This system is a very important component of the body's defenses against infection.

Lymph is a clear colorless fluid, containing cells called lymphocytes and antibodies. Lymph circulates in tiny tubes called lymphatic vessels, or lymphatics. They are present throughout the body and serve as a transport system for invading organisms, which are collected in the lymph nodes. Lymph nodes are structures containing leukocytes, (white blood cells). Leukocytes can engulf and destroy invading organisms and also manufacture antibodies. They will be discussed more fully in the chapter on the blood.

When an infection is present the lymph nodes enlarge in their effort to combat the organisms. They are easily felt in the neck when combating a throat infection.

The tonsils, being visible through the mouth, can be seen to enlarge during an infection of the pharynx. They sometimes remain permanently enlarged because of frequent episodes of pharyngitis in childhood.

A bit of incidental intelligence is that in previous generations it was the custom to remove tonsils from all children because of the notion that they harbored permanent sources of infection. Fortunately, that custom no longer prevails. Tonsils are now removed only if they become so enlarged that they cause pressure on the structures of the nasopharynx, causing ear and sinus infections.

This brings us to the nasopharynx, the place where the nose and throat come together. The disorders that are most likely to occur here are infections that have extended from the nose and/or the throat. Nasopharyngitis is more likely to be of bacterial origin than are infections of the nose or throat. Fevers, earaches, and blowing out pus-containing, (purulent) mucus usually are signs of nasopharyngitis. The appearance of those sighs is a good time to contact your doctor for help.

One thing to keep in mind is that tumors can occur in any organ of the body. They may be cancerous (malignant), or non-cancerous (benign). Any persistent disorder of the pharynx or nasopharynx should be suspected of being malignant. Cancer of a tonsil is not a rare condition, and is a very serious disease.

As we travel a little deeper we encounter the larynx, which is the area of the vocal cords. Most of us have experienced laryngitis, which is usually an infectious process, most often caused by a viral organism, occasionally by bacteria and occasionally due to allergy. Hoarseness is usually the first symptom of laryngitis. If the symptoms are mild it is safe to treat this condition at home, with warm gargles, and sore throat lozenges. Again, if hoarseness with or without serious pain persists beyond a reasonable period, (an elastic period of time, depending on the individual) it's best to call your doctor, or to go in for an examination.

One condition that is seen commonly in singers and in people who shout a lot is called "nodules" on the vocal cords. That condition is actually scarring and thickening of one or both vocal cords. It causes persistent hoarseness, change of voice and loss of control in singing. That condition is remediable with surgery. Persistent hoarseness can also be a sign of cancer of a vocal cord, and should be investigated, preferably by a specialist in head and neck disorders.

The Epiglottis

The epiglottis is a particularly dangerous place for infection in infants and young children. Acute epiglottis, most often due to a viral infection, causes swelling of the airway, sometimes to the extent of asphyxiation.

If an infant shows difficulty breathing, especially if there is a rasping, or squeaking sound with each breath, I would advise calling 911 first, then notify your doctor. If the system works properly the infant will be taken to the closest pediatric emergency room, where emergency treatment can be given to provide an airway. Perhaps your doctor will be in the E.R. when the infant arrives, but usually E.R. physicians are better equipped to handle such a dire emergency.

The same advice applies to the next level down of infection. Acute tracheobronchitis is commonly called CROUP. Croup is a life-threatening emergency. Both croup and acute epiglottis can arise very suddenly in young children without special warning. The first sign of trouble may be a child struggling for breath and wheezing and squeaking. Do not delay in calling 911 IMMEDIATELY. While waiting for the ambulance it can be very helpful to allow the child to breathe steam, either while being held in a shower, or by the close application of a vaporizer. Both acute epiglottis and croup require hospital care to avert a tragedy. Often the emergency state will be ended quickly by prompt good care and the child can go home on the next day.

The Bronchi

Going deeper into the respiratory system we are in the area of the bronchial passages, bronchi). Inflammation of the bronchi, whether due to allergy or infection is called "bronchitis." There is swelling of the mucosal lining of the bronchial passages and spasm of the muscle layer of the bronchi, causing restriction of the airway. There is also increased secretion of mucus, which is consistent with the process of inflammation.

The patient is usually agitated because of severe shortness of breath.

Asthmatic bronchitis (asthma) is defined as reversible obstruction of the bronchial airway. It is most often due to an allergic reaction, caused by presence of an allergen which might be inhaled, ingested, or injected, as in the case of penicillin and some other medications. There is a small incidence of asthma due to purely psychological causes. In most cases it is not possible to identify a specific cause of any given asthmatic attack.

In many cases there is a history of early onset of asthma, often in early childhood. There are also many examples of asthma beginning in mid-life. The attacks are usually acute, meaning that they can begin suddenly and abruptly. When the attacks happen frequently and over a long period of time they can be classed as either chronic asthma or recurrent acute asthma. The outstanding sign of asthma is wheezing and shortness of breath. The sound of a wheeze is like hearing many small pipes, or similar wind instruments, each playing different tones. Wheezing occurs only in the expiratory (exhaling) phase of breathing, not during inspiration, and the expiratory phase is prolonged. There is frequently a cough, productive of thick mucus.

As a general rule asthmatic attacks are not as severe an emergency as acute tracheo-bronchitis (croup), but severe episodes that are not relived promptly can lead to death in many cases. Fortunately, there are many new and effective medications for asthma. The most effective of those are inhaled, and required a prescription. There are some non-prescription medications that can be effective in mild cases of asthma. A good general rule for anyone who has asthma is to be known to a doctor who can give advice and prescribe medications to take early in an attack. Any person who is subject to attacks of asthma should carry an inhaler to dilate the bronchial passages early in the attack. Quite often a person with a severe attack will end up in an emergency room in spite of having a doctor of his own, because emergency rooms are capable of giving more intensive care, and if necessary, admitting the patient to the hospital.

The other kind of bronchitis is due to infection. It is usually slower in onset, but can become as severe as an asthmatic attack if not treated. The infecting organism can be a virus or a bacterium. Both types are usually due to an infection of the upper airway that has extended to the bronchial region. Infectious bronchitis requires treatment to open the bronchial airway, as also does asthma. In most cases of severe infectious bronchitis antibiotic treatment is required to cure the infection, or to prevent a viral infection from being secondarily infected by bacterial organisms. It's good advice to contact your doctor early in the course of bronchitis.

The Alveoli

This region, "the place where the real business of breathing is conducted" can be affected by a number of causes. Physical injuries such as a blow to the chest, possibly with fractured ribs that lacerate the pleural membranes that surround the lungs are not rare. Those occur especially in auto accidents with steering wheel injuries. That usually causes the lung on the injured side of the chest to collapse due to the loss of negative pressure within the chest cavity. That, of course, is a serious emergency. The patient should be hospitalized immediately for intensive treatment to re-inflate the lung.

Another serious injury to the lung is the inhalation of caustic fumes. That can cause great damage, permanent scarring and loss of function of the lung.

One type of injury to the lung, which is widely publicized and ignored by too many is smoking tobacco. It is a clearly proven fact that tobacco smoking can cause cancer of the lung, which is usually fatal. Tobacco smoking is also the major cause of emphysema and pulmonary fibrosis, which are crippling diseases, often leading to death. Yet, the tobacco industry thrives, and people spend millions on cigarettes. There is certainly truth in Shakespeare's expression, "what fools these mortals be."

Pneumonitis

Infection is a very common form of injury to the lung. The proper medical term for this condition is pneumonitis. The common name is pneumonia. Pneumonitis can be caused by viruses, bacteria, or fungus organisms. The earliest symptoms are usually cough and shortness of breath. The most common sign is an abnormal breath sound, heard in inspiration, rather than expiration, as are the wheezes of asthma. This sound is called "rales." It is a high-pitched bubbling over the site of the pneumonia. The sound of rales sometimes fills the entire chest, in severe pneumonitis. It can be heard with a stethoscope or by simply putting ones ear to the chest. There is also dullness to the percussion note—when the chest is thumped with a rigid finger, instead of the usual resonance of a lung filled with air it is a flat high-pitched sound. That is because of the 'itis' in pneumonitis. The air sacs fill with fluid in the site of the infection, causing them to lose their normal resonance.

Chest X-Rays are usually taken as part of the diagnostic workup. It is quite common for no abnormal finding to be seen in the case of viral pneumonitis. Bacterial pneumonitis, on the other hand, usually causes such fluid congestion of the alveoli that it is seen on X-Rays.

Pneumonitis requires serious, and prompt treatment, and in some cases hospitalization. Antibiotics are usually given, often in the case of suspected viral pneumonitis in order to avert bacterial invasion of the infection site. In most cases there is complete recovery without significant scarring of the lungs. If not treated properly, or in the case of individuals whose resistance is severely compromised by some other disease state, pneumonitis can lead to death. In years past, before the advent of antibiotics and our modern effective forms of treatment, pneumonitis was referred to as "the friend of the aged" because it commonly led to death. There is today still a significant incidence of "Pneumonia" as the cause of death of the aged, as a complication of other diseases.

Emphysema

Emphysema is a chronic condition, expected to be present for the lifetime of the patient, rather than the acute conditions that we have discussed thus far. There is abnormal permanent enlargement of the alveolar air spaces with destruction of the walls of the alveoli. It is the end result of chronic lung disease that can be the result of recurrent infections or of the chronic damage caused by tobacco smoking. The patient is chronically short of breath, limited in exercise tolerance and subject to lung infections. There is no curative treatment. Breathing assistance apparatus and supplemental oxygen are frequently required. Surgical removal severely deformed areas of the lung is sometimes required.

Pulmonary Fibrosis

This is a condition of chronic scarring of the lungs with thickening of the walls of the alveoli and loss of the normal elasticity. It is the result of chronic inflammatory conditions, most frequently habitual smoking of cigarettes. Severe recurrent infections, or one of the diseases in the category of "auto-immune diseases" that will be discussed in a later section. The lungs acquire a leathery texture and lose their elasticity. Pulmonary fibrosis is chronic. There is no known cure, and breathing assistance is often needed.

DISORDERS OF THE PLEURA

If a pneumonitis extends to the outermost edge of the lung the infection can involve the pleural membrane that surrounds the lung. The satiny nature of normal pleura enables the lungs to glide outward during inspiration, and inward during expiration. When the pleura is inflamed that membrane becomes red, thickened, and rough. Because the pleura is richly supplied with sensory nerve fibers there is severe pain with each inspiration and each expiration. That condition is called pleuritis, which bears the common name "pleurisy." Accompanying the painful breathing there is a diagnostic sign called the pleural friction rub. It is a rough sandpaper-like sound only heard in the immediate region of the affected pleura with each inspiration and expiration.

It is important to have prompt treatment for relief of the pain, and also the underlying pneumonitis. In most cases there is complete recovery without after-effects if proper treatment is given.

PULMONARY ARTERIAL EMBOLISM

Pulmonary Arterial Embolism is a very serious problem that involves the respiratory and vascular systems. The anatomy and physiology of the cardio-vascular system will be discussed in the next chapter, but in this instance a brief description must be furnished.

An arterial embolus is a clot of blood that lodges in an artery and obstructs the flow of blood through that vessel. In this case the usual origin of the blood clot is a vein in the pelvis, thigh, or leg. It is not uncommon for a leg vein to be injured somehow. As a result of the injury the blood within that vein forms a clot. This often occurs without any pain or sign that the patient might notice. At some point in time a part of the blood clot breaks away from the larger clot and is carried through the veins to the heart. Within the heart venous blood is pumped into the lungs. The blood clot is too large to pass through the vessels of the lungs, and lodges in a narrow artery, blocking that artery completely.

This is a severe medical emergency. The patient is usually thrown into a state of shock. If the clot is large enough to obstruct a major pulmonary artery the patient may die immediately. In many cases it is possible to rescue the patient with intensive acute medical care, but there may be severe permanent damage to the lung.

There are no warning signs or symptoms of an impending pulmonary embolism. In most cases the patient has severe chest pain and collapses. The only proper initial treatment is to CALL 911 IMMEDIATELY.

CANCER OF THE LUNG

The final affliction of the respiratory system to be discussed is cancer. The lungs are prone to cancers which originate within them, and also to cancers which originate in other organs and are carried to the lungs by the blood vessels. As a general rule, cancer of the lung has a particularly poor prognosis in spite of the wonderful modern treatment options for cancer. My only advice to minimize one's chances of having lung cancer is to not begin to smoke, and if you are a smoker, to stop immediately. Of course there are other causes of lung cancer, but smoking cigarettes is clearly considered to be a cause of that deadly disease, and many other diseases.

Smoking is done by choice, so please choose to be a nonsmoker.

There are no identifiable early signs of lung cancer. In most cases the diagnosis is made in the course of an X-Ray taken as part of a routine examination, or in the course of an examination for some other reason. If a suspicious area is seen on X-Ray it usually leads to an extensive workup to identify a possible source of cancer from an organ outside of the lung. If possible, the suspicious site is usually investigated, using one of a number of techniques. Treatment is usually instituted, whether the cancer is primary within the lung or metastatic from some remote location. The statistics for successful cures are quite low.

Tuberculosis and other chronic lung infections constitute a large body of other diseases of the respiratory system, each with its own characteristic symptoms, signs, laboratory findings, treatment and prognosis. In general terms those diseases share the basic characteristics of the ones discussed above and will not be specifically discussed in this book.

There is much more that can be said about the respiratory system but the main objectives of this book have been met. We have discussed the anatomy, physiology, chemistry and the pathology in a brief, but comprehensive way. There is much more information to be had, but this will give the reader a grasp of the fundamentals. We will now go on to the Cardiovascular System.

Chapter Two
THE CARDIOVASCULAR SYSTEM

This system of the body includes the heart and the blood vessels. In the previous chapter we discussed blood vessels including the arteries and arterioles, the veins and the venules, and the capillary beds, the smallest blood vessels that act as an interface between the arterioles and the venules. This chapter will begin with the heart and will include the blood vessels as they fit into the system.

Let's begin by defining and explaining a very important concept from a doctor's point of view: BLOOD PRESSURE. The circulation of blood throughout arteries of the body is driven by a pressure system. The pressure originates in the heart, by its pumping action. The blood pressure is then partially maintained by the pulsations of the arteries, referred to as "the pulse." Blood pressure is measured by a conventional standard in millimeters of mercury. What that means is that amount of pressure required to raise a column of mercury one millimeter. (It's an ancient method of measurement but it has remained as the standard of pressure throughout the world). In the following pages you will see that there are two phases to the beat of the heart; the pumping phase, called the systolic phase, or systole, and the resting phase, called the diastolic phase, or diastole. Blood pressures are expressed as the "systolic" and "diastolic" pressures. An example would be 120/60 meaning that the systolic blood pressure is 120 millimeters of mercury and the diastolic pressure is 60 millimeters of mercury. It is archaic, but it's the standard of practice and it works.

Blood Pressures can be measured anywhere in the body. The most convenient site for measurement is the arm, just above the elbow.

Standards of normal for blood pressure vary with the size and age of the individual. A small child can have a normal blood pressure at 60/40. A small woman could be normal with 90/60. The upper limit of normal for any person has recently been established internationally at 130/80, with slight increase for very large men. There are rumors that the internationally accepted normal will soon be reduced to 120/60 for most people.

Blood pressure can be affected by many factors, such as stress, kidney function, endocrine gland function, loss of volume of circulating blood, as in the case of severe bleeding, and even the amount of salt a person has been taking in. High blood pressure is referred to as hypertension. Low blood pressure is called hypotension. In the case of severe injuries or events such as a heart attack the blood pressure can fall greatly. That person is said to be in a state of shock. High blood pressure is very dangerous because it can cause damage to the heart and many sensitive parts of the body.

ANATOMY AND PHYSIOLOGY OF THE CARDIOVASCULAR SYSTEM

THE HEART

The heart is basically a pump. It is probably the "smartest" pump on earth. The vast bulk of the heart is muscle; surrounding four chambers. For the purpose of explaining the anatomy and physiology the chambers will be called the upper and lower chambers, an oversimplification.

The two upper chambers are called the atria, plural for atrium in Greek, meaning entrance. The lower chambers are the ventricles. The atria have relatively thin walls of muscle, and act mainly as holding chambers. The ventricles, which are the pumps of the heart, have thicker walls. The left ventricle is the main pumping station of the heart. The muscle of the heart is unlike any other muscle in the body. In some areas it is highly modified to resemble nerve tissue and actually conducts electrical impulses in the way that the nerves do, acting as electrical wires.

Now we will trace the pathway of blood through this great pumping station. All the blood in the body, about four to six liters, depending on the size of the person, flows through the heart continuously. The blood enters the heart on its right side (the right-hand side of the body) It is brought to the heart by the largest vein in the body, called the vena cava. The vena cava really consists of two large veins; the inferior vena cava which receives the blood from the lower extremities and the lower part of the body, and the superior vena cava which receives blood from the head and neck, the upper extremities and the upper part of the body. Those large veins merge at the level of the heart to form the Vena Cava. That vein is the final conduit for all the blood returning to the heart from the entire body. It can be one to two inches in diameter depending on the size of the body.

The pumping action of the heart has two phases. The resting phase is called diastole, or the diastolic phase. The phase in which the ventricular muscles contract, pumping the blood, is called systole, or the systolic phase. Blood enters the right atrium during the diastolic phase. About a cupful of blood is immediately passed into the resting right ventricle through a valve that is called the tricuspid valve. Then the systolic phase begins. The tricuspid valve closes, and the right ventricle contracts, squeezing its contents through the pulmonic valve into the lungs. The blood enters the pulmonary artery, and is immediately shunted through a progressively smaller set of arteries and arterioles into the capillary bed of the lungs within the alveolar part of the lung tissue. In the first chapter, the respiratory system, the mechanism of air exchange within the alveoli is explained.

The oxygenated blood then passes into the left atrium, while the heart is still in the diastolic or resting phase. From that chamber it flows through the mitral valve into the left ventricle. Then the ventricles go into the systolic phase. The mitral valve closes and the blood is pushed through the aortic valve, out of the heart, and into the largest blood vessel in the body, the aorta.

We have gone through the pathway followed by the blood through the heart. Now let's examine the heart itself in some detail. The muscle of the heart is greatly specialized. That muscle is amazingly durable, in that it contracts and relaxes 60-80 times every minute in most people every minute of one's life. If we take age 80 as the average lifespan these days, a little arithmetic will show you that that is an amazing number of contractions during a lifespan. I can think of no other muscle that does as much work. Because that pump is so reliable, we rarely think about it until something goes wrong.

The rate of the heart beat is controlled chiefly by the heart itself and in part by events that are going on elsewhere in the body. The pacemaker of a normal heart is located within the heart muscle high in the region of the right atrium. Studies have shown that a specimen of that part of the heart muscle when isolated from the rest of the heart emits an electrical impulse with a continuous regular beat. As was mentioned earlier, some of the muscle fibers of the heart are highly modified to act as electrical wires. They conduct those electrical impulses that originate in a small structure called the sino-atrial node and relay those impulses to another small structure called the atrioventricular node. Those impulses are then carried through the conduction fibers of the heart, called the Purkinje fibers to the ventricular muscles. In response to the stimulus originated and relayed by those centers the muscles contract into the systolic phase, and when the stimulus stops the muscles relax into the diastolic phase. The rate at which those nodes discharge electrical impulses is regulated by the nodes themselves, but is also influenced by messages from the brain, the endocrine organs, chiefly the thyroid gland, and the metabolism of the body tissues.

For the reader who wishes more scientific detail, the opening and closing of the heart valves is controlled by pressure gradients within the chambers of the heart. In the state of diastole the tricuspid valve, leading from the right atrium to the right ventricle is open, allowing blood to enter the right ventricle. The pulmonic valve, which allows blood to flow from the right ventricle into the lungs is closed. The mitral valve, leading from the left atrium into the left ventricle is open, allowing the left ventricle to fill with blood. The aortic valve, leading from the left ventricle to the aorta is closed. The filling of the right atrium, the right ventricle, and the left atrium are all done passively during the diastolic phase. When the chambers contract in systole the build-up of pressure within those chambers causes the tricuspid valve to close, the pulmonic valve to open, the mitral valve to close, and the aortic valve to open. This allows the great squeezing action of the heart to move the blood into the appropriate chambers, and out into the aorta to be distributed throughout the body.

With apologies to those readers whose eyes have glazed over during the detailed description just past, this author must express his great respect for the complexity and the reliability of that great pump, the heart.

Although the heart receives and pumps out all of the blood in the body it cannot use any of that blood for its own needs. The nutrition of the heart muscle and the means of excretion of its waste products are handled by a separate system of vessels called the coronary blood vessels.

An important yet rarely discussed component of the cardiovascular anatomy is the pericardium. That is the sac that envelops the heart. It is actually a continuation of the membrane that envelops the lungs, the pleura. As in the case of the pleura, the pericardium is a fibrous, serous membrane. Its smooth and slippery inner surface enables the movement of the heart within the sac. The pericardium has a thick, tough fibrous outer layer that supports the heart muscle in its contractions. It is a vital part of the heart.

THE ARTERIES

Arteries have walls composed of three layers. The inner layer, called the intima, is thin and smooth, composed of cells called endothelium. The middle layer, called the muscularis layer, is thick and is composed of specialized muscle cells interspersed with an elastic connective tissue. The outer layer, called the adventitia, is a tough sheet of fibrous tissue.

The aorta is the largest artery in the body. It begins at the aortic valve, which is located on the posterior surface of the heart. The aorta travels in an upward, (cephalad) direction, then turns in a sweeping arch to the left, then proceeds in a downward, (caudad) direction. From the ascending portion branch the arteries leading to the coronary arteries, the arms and structures of the chest. From the mid-arch come the arteries to the face, head, and brain. During its downward sweep the aorta gives off the arteries to all of the structures of the chest and abdomen.

At a point several inches below the belly button, (umbilicus) the aorta divides to form the right and left common iliac arteries. Those divide into the internal and external iliac arteries, along the way giving off smaller branches to some of the organs within the abdomen. The internal iliacs go into the pelvic region, supplying the male and female pelvic organs. The external iliac arteries then go through the groin, (inguinal region) where they become the femoral arteries. The femorals then branch into the deep and superficial femoral arteries. The superficial femorals furnish blood to the skin and superficial structures of the legs. The deep femorals, located adjacent to the bones of the legs, provide circulation to the deeper muscles and related structures. The arterial supply to the feet is derived from branches of the femoral arteries.

THE VEINS

Veins are made up of three layers, as are the arteries, but the layers are quite different. The inner layer, also called the intima, is composed of endothelial cells as are found in the arteries. The median layer is much thinner than that of the arteries. Instead of the thick muscular and elastic tissue layer it is quite thin, having some circular muscle fibers in the larger veins and only thin connective tissue in the smaller vessels. The outer layer, the adventitia is composed of fibrous connective tissue, but is much thinner than that of the arteries. Some veins, specifically those of the lower extremities have valves located at intervals.

The veins are the vessels that receive blood from all parts of the body, and return that blood to the heart. The veins also receive metabolic products from the liver and pancreas and all the endocrine glands. That blood is rich in nutrients and metabolic products, such as hormones from the endocrine glands, and also waste products that the veins return to the heart. The heart then sends the blood to the arteries to be transported to the kidneys and liver for excretion of waste products and also to carry nutrition to all parts of the body.

Because the veins carry blood toward the heart we will begin our tour of the veins at the toes and fingers. In the toes blood is transferred via the capillary beds from the arterioles to the venules. Those enter larger veins, which flow into the counterparts of the femoral arteries, the deep and superficial saphenous veins. Just below, (distal to) the inguinal regions the superficial saphenous vein empties into the deep femoral vein in each leg, becoming the femoral veins. Just inside the abdomen the femoral veins flow into the internal and external iliac veins, which then flow into the common iliac veins. The common iliac veins then flow into the inferior vena cava, carrying that blood toward the heart.

As the inferior vena cava progresses toward the heart it is joined by tributary veins, bringing blood from all of the abdominal organs and from the adjacent muscles and other structures to be returned to the heart. When the inferior vena cava reaches the heart it joins the superior vena cava. The combined great veins then join to return the blood via the vena cava into the right atrium.

THE PHYSIOLOGY OF THE ARTERIES AND THE VEINS

Arteries carry blood away from the heart to supply every part of the body. There is a measurable pressure within all arteries because they are part of the pumping force that drives the blood throughout the body. Veins, on the other hand, carry blood back to the heart passively. They do not have any measurable pressure within their lumen.

Arteries play a very active role in the conduction of blood. They assist in the propulsion of blood through their lumen by their ability to generate a pulse wave. Pulses are easily felt in the neck, the wrists, and in parts of the arms and legs. The pulse wave begins in the aorta which receives its blood from the strong systolic squeezing force of the left ventricle of the heart. When that cupful of blood slams into the aorta that artery receives the blood in its relaxed (diastolic) phase, and fills with the blood. Then the muscularis layer of the aorta recoils, and contracts, pushing the blood to the next segment of artery. That pulsation is continued throughout all of the arteries and arterioles. The arterial pulsation is remarkably rhythmic, serving to propel the blood away from the heart to all parts of the body. In the capillaries there is no pulsation. The blood flows into the venules and the veins passively.

Veins do not have any pulsation in the normal state of health. They carry blood passively, assisted by the body's muscular contractions, and partly by the force of gravity. One can easily see the difference between arterial and venous bleeding by observing the bleeding from a laceration. If an artery is cut the blood comes forth in spurts, pushed out by the pulse wave. Venous bleeding, by contrast is a steady, smooth flow without spurting. Blood loss from the laceration of a large vein can be very severe, but the spurting of blood from a large artery is much more rapid. Both require immediate care to stop the bleeding and to repair the laceration.

Capillary bleeding can be seen in the case of a surface abrasion of the skin. There is a mild, slow oozing of blood which can usually be stopped with local pressure over the bleeding site.

DISORDERS OF THE CARDIOVASCULAR SYSTEM

"It's been happening for a while, but it seems to be bothering me more, so I came in to see you, doctor. I feel a shaking or quivering in my chest. At first it came and went, but lately it has been there all the time. I get tired and short of breath more easily. My appetite is good and I've been sleeping OK, but I'm beginning to worry about it." Physical examination showed the blood pressure to be normal. The heart rate was about 80 per minute, but the rhythm was found to be irregular. An EKG revealed atrial fibrillation as the rhythm. Because of his age (75), and the fact that his heart otherwise tested out to be normal, and in view of the fact that his abnormal heart rhythm had been present for several months the decision was made to not attempt to convert his cardiac rhythm to normal, but to give him medication to keep his heart rate at the present level or lower and to observe him at intervals. He has done well for more than a year.

(Illustration Case)

DISORDERS OF THE HEART

Let's begin this discussion with a classical case of "heart attack." That most often means sudden blockage of a coronary artery that supplies oxygen and nutrition to the muscle of the heart. It is usually labeled a "coronary heart attack" or a "Coronary." There is quite often a warning symptom that precedes a coronary heart attack. It's important to look at that first.

Angina

The correct medical name for it is "angina pectoris." That name refers to a very particular kind of chest pain. The pain of angina is often described as a "heavy sensation", or "squeezing pain." Angina is usually felt in the left side of the chest, sometimes very low in the chest, or even in the upper abdomen. The pain usually radiates upward, frequently into the neck or jaws. It often goes to the left shoulder and sometimes radiates down the left arm. It is often accompanied by sweating. True pain of angina usually subsides in five minutes or less. If the pain lasts for a significantly longer period it is likely that a true coronary heart attack is taking place. Angina very frequently, but not always, occurs and recurs, but is ignored over a long period of time. It often gets worse, reaching a crescendo before the coronary heart attack finally occurs. Angina is frequently dismissed as "indigestion" by a patient who denies the possibility of having real heart pain. It's really important to pay attention to any chest pain and to believe that it could be a warning message. That could save your life.

A Coronary Heart Attack

In our anatomical tour we saw that the heart receives its own blood supply from a special set of arteries called the coronary arteries. Those arteries originate from small openings in the region of the aortic valve, providing oxygenated blood and nutrients to nourish the heart muscle. The coronary arteries are susceptible to the disease process called atherosclerosis, which is the proper medical term for the more common word "arteriosclerosis." Atherosclerosis is discussed in detail in a later section on diseases of the arteries.

So, we start with a condition of atherosclerotic plaque formation within the intima of the coronary arteries. The plaque may be thick enough to partially occlude the coronary artery. The most modern theory is that there is also an underlying inflammatory or infectious change in the intima of the artery, causing the intima and its plaque to become brittle and fragile. Then a section of plaque breaks loose at its upstream edge, due to the pressure of the flow of blood, and flips up, blocking the passage of blood beyond that point.

Because the blood flow stops, a blood clot, (thrombus) is formed at the site of the obstruction. The thrombus extends downstream of the obstruction, causing obstruction of smaller branches. A part of the heart muscle is deprived of its blood supply. Because heart muscle has a very high demand for oxygen and other nutrients from the blood the muscle that is deprived of its blood begins to die almost immediately. The medical term for this event is myocardial, (heart muscle), infarction, (death due to loss of blood supply). In typical doctor shorthand, that is abbreviated to M.I.

That is the underlying part of what often happens in a heart attack. The events of a M.I. are severely shocking to the heart. Sometimes the heart simply stops beating, and the patient dies instantly. In most cases that does not happen. The shock to the heart often causes it to lose its normal rhythm and to beat abnormally. That is called a state of arrhythmia. The rate of the heart might become very rapid, because of a condition called atrial fibrillation or another type of tachyarrhythmia (rapid arrhythmia), or it might become very slow (bradyarrhythmia) because of a blockage of the normal electrical conduction through the internal conduction system of the heart. In either case the patient often loses consciousness, and is unable to help himself or herself.

If the patient is lucky, someone will call 911. Again, if luck prevails, help will arrive quickly in the form of paramedics who have the capability to attend to the patient's immediate needs and if supreme good luck holds out the patient will be taken to a hospital E.R. that is capable of diagnosing the problem and treating it. Arrhythmia will be corrected, the blood pressure will be restored to normal and most likely, the patient will be given anticoagulant medication to stop the progression of the thrombosis and save as much heart muscle as possible. Then the patient will be transferred to the heart catherization laboratory for internal examination of the coronary arteries and emergency treatment. Then he or she will be transferred to an Intensive Care Unit for close monitoring and treatment.

If good emergency care can be obtained quickly there is a fair chance that the patient will make a good recovery if the initial M.I. was not so disastrous as to destroy too much heart muscle.

That is a reasonably accurate account of the events that constitute a coronary heart attack. Of course, the very technical details, such as the stepwise development of atherosclerosis, and the events of the formation of a thrombus have been omitted, but will be discussed in further sections of the book.

Heart Failure

The proper full name for this condition is CONGESTIVE HEART FAILURE, (CHF). It is a condition that occurs when the ability of the heart to pump blood into the arteries to be distributed throughout the body falls behind the volume of blood being returned to the heart via the venous system. The most common circumstances causing CHF are severe overload of fluid volume within the circulating blood plasma and/or pump failure of the heart.

Increase in the volume of fluid circulating within the blood vessels can be due to either an increase in the volume of fluid taken into and held by the body, or a decrease in the ability of the body to excrete the proper volume of circulating fluids. A very common example of the first is that of a person who takes in a great excess of salt in his/her diet. In order for the body to retain that salt it must provide a certain volume of water that will hold the salt in solution. Salt overload is very common in the everyday lives of most of us. We then become thirsty and drink more water or any available liquid. If our urinary system works well we will produce more urine and be able to excrete the excess fluid and salt in our urine. If we have a severe problem such as diseased kidneys that cannot concentrate the urine in order to excrete the salt, or some endocrine abnormality that prevents proper stimulation of the kidneys to increase their work load, or a severe obstruction of the outflow of urine that allows a backing-up of pressure within the urinary system, then fluid overload occurs.

On the other side of the coin, if we have a dysfunctional heart, whether due to severe valvular disease that causes enlargement and weakness of the left ventricle, or an abnormal heart rhythm that causes very rapid and weak pumping action, or very slow pumping action the pump will fail.

When, for either reason, the heart begins to fail to pump out the blood that is being returned via the venous system the effect is first noted in the lungs. The pressure in the veins, building up throughout the body is increased within the venules of the alveolar exchange system. The walls of the capillaries distend, stretching to the point at which fluid from the plasma leaks into the alveolar air spaces, displacing the space needed for air exchange. Rales become audible throughout the chest. The result is shortness of breath and more rapid rate of respirations. Oxygenation of the blood is diminished greatly and the patient's entire body suffers from oxygen deprivation. Also, the rate of clearance of waste gases from the blood suffers, and those products, toxic in nature, accumulate. If not corrected, that cycle can lead to the death of the patient.

Other very serious effects of congestive heart failure are severe congestion of the vascular system of the liver, interfering with normal liver function, and passive congestion of all organs of the body. A very easily seen sign of vascular congestion is edema, the accumulation of fluid in the tissues close to the skin. There can be severe swelling of the legs, feet and hands, and puffiness of the eyes and cheeks.

Congestive heart failure is a very common disorder and a very frequent cause of hospitalization. If not treated properly it can lead to death. It is very important that the cause of CHF be accurately determined and corrected if possible. Treatment might require heart surgery or placing the patient on some form of cardiac medication to control an abnormal rhythm, or some form of dialysis to support diseased kidneys. This disorder can usually be diagnosed correctly and in most cases helpful treatment can be given provided a complete and correct diagnosis is made.

Cardiac Arrhythmias

The term "cardiac arrhythmia" means abnormal rhythm of the heart. A heart that has been beating regularly for many years can suddenly lose its regular rhythm due to some event, either in the heart itself, or in another organ that has an effect on the heart. An example of the former would be a coronary heart attack that damages a part of the heart that regulates the rhythm. The latter would be exemplified by hyperthyroidism, a state of over-activity of the thyroid gland causing over-production of thyroid hormone. That condition causes the heart to beat rapidly.

Excessively rapid heart rate is called tachycardia. Excessively slow rate is called bradycardia. Either of those rates can cause severe alteration in the function of the heart.

The most commonly encountered arrhythmia is called atrial fibrillation. That is a rapid and irregular heartbeat originating in the atria of the heart. The most lethal arrhythmias are called ventricular tachycardia and ventricular fibrillation. In those arrhythmias the ventricles of the heart beat very rapidly, independently of atrial function. The result can be sudden death due to a coronary heart attack or congestive heart failure due to loss of normal pumping action of the heart.

Arrhythmias are treated with medications, electrical shocking of the heart and electrical pacing of the heart by artificial pacemakers. Medications are given either on an acute, temporary basis or for permanent stabilization of the rhythm. Electrical shocking is done using external shocking devices, usually to stop ventricular arrhythmias. The electrical shock usually causes the heart to stop beating briefly, stopping the ventricular arrhythmia. Then, in most cases, the heart resumes a normal rhythm. If not, external heart pacing is instituted. Electrical pacing of the heart is done either with external pacemakers, or for permanent chronic use by means of a small battery driven pacing unit that is inserted within the chest wall of the patient with wires implanted into the heart muscle, delivering a small, regular electrical impulse to maintain a regular heart beat. Modern permanent implanted pacemakers can also have a shocking feature that automatically shocks the heart internally in the event of ventricular arrhythmias. Bradycardia is best treated with a permanently implanted pacemaker that can respond to sudden slowing of the rate of the heart and correct the bradycardia by delivering a regular stimulating impulse to the heart at a proper rate.

A very important fact is that the state of the art in the treatment of arrhythmias has advanced greatly over the past twenty- five years. If a patient can be treated promptly in a competent medical facility there is a good chance of rescuing most people with arrhythmias, and extending their lives for many years.

Valvular Heart Disease

Disease of the heart valves is another type of serious heart disorder. It is imperative for normal heart performance to have properly functioning heart valves. There are three major causes of diseased heart valves. The first is congenital absence or malformation of one or more valves. This is detectable at birth by the appearance of the baby and by conspicuously abnormal heart sounds. In one type of birth defect the blood is not properly oxygenated when it enters the circulation and the oxygen-poor blood causes a bluish discoloration of the skin. That bluish discoloration is called "cyanosis", commonly referred to as a "blue baby." That defect can be remedied by a delicate operation, usually performed by a pediatric cardiac surgeon. The results are most often successful. Unfortunately, there are often multiple other birth defects associated with congenital heart disorders, some of which are very serious. There are other types of congenital deformities of the heart. Some can be corrected surgically, and others, sadly, cannot.

Another kind of valvular heart disease is that caused by rheumatic fever and other related inflammatory disorders. In the course of those diseases one or more of the four valves is often attacked by the inflammatory process of the disease, which results in scarring of the valve. That scarring can deform the valve so that it cannot function normally. In many cases that kind of valvular disease can be corrected surgically.

A third kind of valvular heart disease is that which occurs as the result of disease of the heart muscle. A good example is that caused by hypertension, (high blood pressure). That condition often stretches the aorta at the point of attachment of the aortic valve, causing incomplete closure of the aortic valve in diastole. That condition is referred to as "aortic insufficiency." That causes back- flow of blood into the left ventricle after systolic emptying of that chamber. The result is further enlargement of the left ventricle and hypertrophic change in the muscle wall of the left ventricle.

If a heart valve becomes damaged by scarring, as in the case of an inflammatory disorder the results can be obstruction of the flow of blood through that valve. That condition is referred to as "stenosis" of the valve, which means narrowing of the passageway. If the valve becomes incompetent because of stretching of its attachments, or because of scarring that prevents the valve from closing completely that condition is referred to as "insufficiency" of the valve, in Doctor Speak. In either case; valvular stenosis or insufficiency, there is usually a surgical remedy, replacing the diseased valve with an artificial valve or with a pig's heart valve. Both of those choices are routinely offered.

Another kind of problem that can seriously affect the function of the heart valves is rupture of the tiny muscles and tendons that control the active part of opening of the heart valve. That is usually due to wear and tear on those muscles and tendons. When that happens abruptly the patient usually experiences an immediate change in breathing and in exercise tolerance. The change can be mild, or so severe as to cause immediate collapse.

Surgical repair and replacement of diseased heart valves is now an everyday procedure at most major medical centers. The heart is stopped, and the circulation of blood throughout the body is maintained by a heart-lung pump that oxygenates and circulates the blood. With the heart stopped the surgeon can examine and repair the valve, or remove the diseased valve and select a replacement valve to sew into its place. In most cases the patient notices immediate improvement after that surgery. Replacement valves sometimes need to be replaced, depending on the longevity of the patient. Valve replacement is a routine surgical procedure today.

The technique of stopping the heart and using a heart-lung bypass pump is routine today for the correction of valvular defects and coronary artery disease.

Diseases Of The Heart Muscle

Earlier in this chapter there was a description of the disease process called myocardial infarction. That is a disease state caused by interruption of the blood supply to a part of the heart muscle due to blockage of one or more coronary arteries. It is a permanent state, because the area of damaged muscle heals into a scar that cannot contract or relax in the manner of normal myocardial tissue.

There are other kinds of diseases of the muscle of the heart muscle that are not rare, and are very serious. The two most commonly seen are myocarditis and cardiomyopathy. Myocarditis is an acute inflammatory state. The cause in nearly all cases is infection, most commonly by a viral organism. In that disease the heart is attacked by a virus, usually as an extension of a generalized viral infection elsewhere in the body. The effect on the heart muscle is frequently devastating. Large areas of the heart muscle become inflamed. When that happens, the performance of the heart as a pump is severely affected. The patient becomes short of breath and sometimes loses consciousness. In severe cases there is death unless the patient can be treated in a state of the art cardiac care center. The after-effect of the acute infection, if the patient survives the initial damage, is permanent loss of adequate heart function. In that case heart transplantation might be the only remedy. There are certainly many instances of acute myocarditis that are not as devastating, but in most cases the patient is very sick, requiring hospital care for some times long periods of time.

The second condition, cardiomyopathy, is usually a chronic process, rather than an acute one. It is due to ongoing injury to the heart, most frequently by the ingestion of toxic substances. Alcoholic cardiomyopathy ranks very high on the list of causes. Chronic alcoholics have a particular predisposition to this disease which dominates the state of their health more than the usual liver dysfunction. Cardiomyopathy and liver disease often exist concurrently. This disorder can also occur as the result of an auto-immune disease involving the entire body, such as those in the rheumatic fever family of diseases. The end result is the same. The heart muscle becomes flabby and weak. There is gradual progression of shortness of breath and general swelling of the body due to salt and water retention, leading to death in severe cases. Patients with this disorder are usually poor candidates for heart transplantation because of the severe deterioration of other systems of the body.

Cancer of the heart muscle is so extremely rare that it will be mentioned only as a rare disease of the heart.

DISORDERS OF THE BLOOD VESSELS

DISEASES OF THE ARTERIES

There are four main categories of arterial diseases: atherosclerotic disease, congenital malformations, thromboembolic events, and inflammatory diseases. We will discuss atherosclerotic disease, the most common disease, last, and will begin with congenital disorders.

Congenital Disorders of the Arteries

The most sinister congenital problem of the arteries is arterial aneurysm. That name is given to an artery that has a weak spot from the time of birth. Unfortunately, many congenital aneurysms occur in the arteries of the brain. There is rarely any advance symptom to warn of the existence of a cerebral aneurysm before it ruptures. Rupture frequently occurs in a person in the twenties or thirties. The results can be devastating. Blood under pressure is released from the artery and goes freely into very soft and sensitive brain tissue, usually inflicting severe and permanent damage. In a fortunate few there are headaches or neurologic symptoms caused by the enlarging aneurysm that bring the patient to a doctor. If the doctor is intelligent and well-trained he or she will be concerned enough to refer the patient to a neurologist or neurosurgeon immediately. By means of modern imaging techniques the aneurysm can be detected before it ruptures. Some sort of surgical procedure will follow and the patient will be spared any serious damage. Modern surgical repair of aneurysms is really very good. If there is no warning or if the warning is unheeded the results can be tragic.

Aneurysms of arteries also occur as the result of atherosclerotic degeneration. These can be in any artery within the body and constitute a serious problem if they are of sufficient size to be in the "likely to rupture" category. This is especially true of aneurysms of the thoracic and abdominal portions of the aorta. Surgical repair of those aneurysms is difficult, but can be successfully done in qualified surgical centers, generally with good results.

There is one specific type of aneurysm that deserves special description. That is dissecting aneurysm of the thoracic portion of the aorta, caused by rupture of an atherosclerotic plaque within the intima. The aorta carries the greatest pressure of any artery. It has a three -layered construction, as do all other arteries. The median and adventitia layers are much thicker than in other arteries. If a break occurs in the intimal layer blood under very high pressure can flow into the median layer. There is immediate distention with blood between the layers of the aorta. That distention can in some cases be only for a short segment, or can extend throughout the entire length of the aorta. That distortion of the lumen can shut off the flow of blood to all the arterial branches in the involved segment of the aorta.

Dissecting aneurysm of the aorta is frequently fatal. Only prompt and skillful surgical intervention can save the life of the patient. Many people are saved due to good surgery and most patients, after a prolonged period of convalescence, can return to moderate activity.

There can be aneurysmal dilatation of any artery anywhere in the body. Aneurysms of the abdominal portion of the aorta are quite common. It is fortunate that most of those can be detected early by the symptoms they cause or by their appearance. Surgical repair of aneurysms of the abdominal aorta is quite often successful in the hands of an experienced vascular surgeon. If there is rupture of an arterial aneurysm outside of the brain there is a good chance that it can be corrected surgically.

Another congenital arterial disorder, not commonly seen, is called Arterio-venous malformation. In that condition there is direct connection between an artery and a vein, instead of the usual transition from arterioles to capillaries to venules to veins. That is a very serious disorder and a frequent cause of death.

Thromboembolic Disease

The name refers to the condition in which a blood clot, (thrombus) is released into the circulation and is carried through progressively smaller vessels until it lodges in an artery that is too small to allow it to pass, thereby blocking any further blood flow through that vessel.

The great majority of thrombi that enter the arterial circulation originate in the veins of the leg or the pelvis. That is the chief source of pulmonary emboli, discussed in the previous chapter. Now we will concern ourselves with thrombi that originate in the heart, and are passed into the general circulation.

Thrombi of cardiac origin begin in the left atrium of the heart. There is in most people a small pocket called the atrial appendage, or auricle, within the left atrium. This is a common site of eddy currents in the blood passing through the left atrium. The tumbling of blood in that appendage sometimes causes the blood to remain static within the appendage, leading to the formation of a thrombus. That blood clot is semi-solid. If it leaves the left atrium it enters the left ventricle and is pushed out of the heart and enters the aorta. The thrombus then can enter any convenient artery. If the artery is one leading to the brain the thrombus eventually lodges in a smaller artery within the brain, blocking any further blood flow through that artery. That is a cerebral thrombosis. Brain tissue has a very high demand for oxygen. The affected tissue can die. It is the most frequent cause of stroke.

Emboli can also pass into the arteries going to the abdominal organs and to the legs. If the embolus lodges in an arterial branch supplying one of the abdominal viscera or in a major artery in a leg there can be severe damage due to loss of blood supply. In such a case emergency surgery is required to restore the circulation to the affected part.

Inflammatory Disease of the Arteries

The proper name for that type of condition is "arteritis", true to our convention of labeling inflammatory conditions. Arteritis is in the general family of auto-immune diseases. The cause is unknown. When an artery becomes diseased with arteritis the intimal lining and sub-intima become greatly swollen. The degree of thickening can be so great that the artery is completely blocked, preventing any flow of blood. Thick scar tissue can form in the inflamed vessels.

Although any artery can be affected by this condition, one artery has a specific tendency for acute arteritis. That is the temporal artery whose pulsations can be felt easily in the temples on either side of the head. Temporal arteritis is most often accompanied by severe and persistent headache and tenderness on the affected side of the head in the region of the temple. That artery sends a branch to the retina of the eye. If the lumen of that branch becomes blocked it can lead to blindness in the affected eye. Treatment of the arteritis with steroid medication usually averts blindness if the condition is diagnosed and treated early enough, before complete obstruction can occur.

Arteritis can occur in any artery in the body. Early and aggressive care is always necessary.

Atherosclerosis

This is a topic that has been of concern to the medical community worldwide for some time. It is all about cholesterol and heart attacks and strokes.

Nutritionists and manufacturers of dietary supplements are busy designing diets and manufacturing and selling products to help, but there has been quite a lot of change in the way some of our best cardiologists and research scientists look at the causes of coronary heart attacks and strokes. I will attempt to lay out the traditional view of atherosclerosis and will cite the "new ideas" as I know them to be.

Atherosclerosis is a condition in which there is deposition of fatty material, chiefly made from circulating cholesterol together with calcium and other materials, within the lumen of arteries.

The nature of those deposits of material, located just beneath the intimal layer of arteries, is the subject of much study and discussion among doctors at the present time. For many years the theory was that cholesterol simply deposited in the arteries in a gradual manner, slowly building up a layer thick enough to block the lumen of the artery. This kind of blockage would be exactly like the blockage of plumbing pipes after years of usage.

Current theory is based on scientific investigation done through angiography. That is a technique of visualizing the inside of arteries by inserting very small tubes, (catheters) into the artery, injecting a substance which shows on X-Ray, and taking pictures and small biopsy samples from the intima and subintima with that catheter.

The current thinking about the cause of obstruction of the coronary arteries is that in addition to the presence of too much cholesterol in the blood there has to be some type of injury to the intima. Infection is one theory of possible injury, and inflammation caused by an auto-immune process is being investigated.

Coronary artery obstruction is most commonly treated by a surgical procedure called coronary artery bypass grafting. In that surgery small tubes of synthetic material are used to bypass the obstructed portion of the coronary artery and are sewn as a bridge connecting the unobstructed portion of the artery with its point of entry in the heart. It is very common that multiple coronary arteries are found to be obstructed. In that case multiple bypasses are done. There is a very high rate of success with that procedure, greatly extending the life of the patient.

It is comforting to know that coronary artery bypass surgery is there and that it is quite successful and available in most large communities, but it would be much more comforting to know a way to PREVENT coronary artery disease. Research into new medications and diets is going on throughout the world. I feel that there is reason to expect that some good answers and solutions will eventually be found. In the meanwhile I continue to strongly advise that everyone assumes the responsibility of taking care of oneself. Eat sensibly to bring your weight within the healthy, normal range. Exercise regularly, Do Not Smoke! See your doctor regularly and do your best to deal with stress and anxiety in these stressful times.

DISORDERS OF THE VEINS

Venous Thrombosis and Thrombophlebitis

Thrombi can occur within arteries, as seen in the previous section, or within veins. Venous thrombosis is much more common than arterial thrombosis. The chief reason for that is that blood flows more slowly within veins than within arteries. There is no pulsing action and there is no pressure within veins.

When blood stands still for long periods of time it has a tendency to clot. The flow of blood through the veins of the lower extremities is greatly enhanced by the pumping action of the muscles surrounding the veins. When one remains in a fixed position for any length of time, as in a long trip in an airplane or an automobile, that pumping action is absent and the blood moves very slowly or not at all. The medical term for that is "venous stasis."

Venous stasis promotes the formation of venous thrombi. This is particularly true of patients in the post-operative state. They are unable to move, or are discouraged from moving because of their surgery. There is also a significant risk for the aged, who nay sit still for long periods of time. For that reason hospital recovery rooms routinely provide long tight stockings for their post-operative patients. Hospital patients who are unable to move for long periods of time are given pneumatic stockings that perform a sequential squeezing action on the legs to keep venous blood moving.

In the first chapter on the respiratory system we detailed the events and the destructive effect of a pulmonary artery embolus. Keep in mind that the thrombus that was thrown from the right ventricle into the pulmonary artery most likely began as a venous thrombosis in a leg or pelvic vein.

Superficial Thrombophlebitis

If a thrombosis occurs in a superficial vein in the leg, especially if that vein is diseased with varicosis, an inflammatory process occurs. The vein becomes enlarged, the overlying skin becomes reddened and warm, and the patient has pain. That condition is called thrombophlebitis. Thrombophlebitis in a superficial leg vein is easily seen and felt through the skin. There often is local redness overlying the affected vein, accompanied by tenderness. In most cases superficial thrombophlebitis is self-limited, stopping short of becoming a major problem. However, if the thrombophlebitis is in the thigh, and continues to ascend toward the groin the situation becomes serious. Quite often a surgical procedure is necessary to tie off the affected superficial saphenous vein, preventing the thrombus from entering the deep femoral vein, to then be carried to the heart.

Deep Vein Thrombosis

Deep vein thrombosis is quite a different problem and usually a much more serious one. The deep leg veins have a direct pipeline access to the femoral vein and therefore to the vena cava. They are located deep within the leg, usually close to the bones. If a thrombosis occurs in a deep vein there is usually a deep ache within the leg, and only a mild swelling of the calf, and in some cases, puffy swelling of the ankle. There is some calf tenderness that can be very slight. There may or may not be some reddish discoloration of the overlying skin. In addition to the calf tenderness there is often but not always another physical sign: if the foot is stretched upward the calf muscles are tightened and there is some pull on the calf veins. That causes pain in most but not all patients. That is called Homanns' sign.

There is a reliable diagnostic test for the presence of this potentially serious thrombosis, called the duplex scan. It is a non-invasive, inexpensive test, using a doppler ultrasound instrument. Most physicians will order that test immediately after seeing the patient. If the test is positive the patient is often hospitalized immediately for bed rest and treatment with an anticoagulant medication to stop the propagation of the thrombus. If deep venous thrombosis is not detected in time a piece of the thrombus can break loose and embolize to the lung. Pulmonary embolization can be a disastrous event, causing instant death. In most cases, however, that condition responds to treatment. In any case there can be severe permanent damage to the lung.

Varicose Veins

All leg veins have small valves distributed throughout their length. The effect of those tiny valves is to retard the blood within the vein from obeying the law of gravity and settling downward. In many people, chiefly because of a congenital predisposition, those valves fail. The veins become distended with blood and become permanently stretched. The swelling of the veins is called "varicosity" and the veins are called varicose veins. Varicose veins are a common complication of pregnancy. That is because the enlargement of the uterus causes pressure on the leg veins, slowing the return of blood and distending the veins. Actually, veins in other parts of the body can become varicosed, but they are not as conspicuous as most of the leg veins.

Varicose veins of the leg are very common. They are routinely treated as cosmetic problems. The large veins can be removed surgically and the small "spider veins" are treated by injection or laser therapy.

THE DIVERSE FUNCTIONS OF THE BLOOD VESSELS

We have finished our tour of the cardiovascular system, but it is important to look at the inter-relationship between the blood vessels and other parts of the body. Only two major systems, the nervous system and the blood vessels have such a wide-reaching effect on virtually every part of the body. It is a fair statement that if there is a breakdown in either of those systems it will be felt throughout the entire body.

No part of the body can function normally without healthy arteries and veins. If any part of the skin is deprived of its circulation it will break down. Skin ulcers will form and will not heal without medical help. If any vital organ loses its circulation due to arterial obstruction from atherosclerosis or blockage of an artery from an embolus that organ will be seriously compromised and if untreated will probably die. That means that the patient could die from that organ failure unless it is corrected.

The name given to failure of an organ due to loss of blood supply is "gangrene." Two good examples are loss of blood supply to a leg, and to a section of the intestine. In the first instance there is a very common history of a gradual loss of circulation to a leg due to the slow formation of atherosclerosis blocking a major artery. The patient usually experiences cramping of the calf muscles of the affected leg when walking. That pain is called "intermittent claudication." Claudication is the equivalent pain to angina, the pain from the heart muscle due to inadequate blood supply. Angina is a warning that there could be a coronary heart attack unless some type of interventional treatment is given. In the case of intermittent claudication that pain is a warning that there is serious blockage of an artery that supplies blood to that leg. Usually, if medical help is sought in time, the blockage can be located and corrected by some sort of surgical procedure.

In the case of blockage of an artery that supplies a part of the intestine there is usually no advance warning. The artery becomes blocked and thrombus forms very soon thereafter. Because the arteries that supply the intestine are carried in tissue called the mesentery, that event is called a mesenteric artery thrombosis. The result is immediate abdominal pain that becomes more severe rapidly. A segment of intestine becomes gangrenous and dies. Unless surgery is performed soon the patient will die. Usually the gangrenous segment of the intestine can be removed and the intestine re-connected and the patient survives. That really depends on the prompt intervention of a skilled surgeon.

This scenario can be repeated with loss of blood supple to any part of the body. The more vital the part affected, the greater the necessity for prompt and expert care. The take-home lesson here is that no part of the body can live without a good blood supply.

Chapter Three
THE DIGESTIVE SYSTEM

At the beginning of the first chapter I stated that problems of the respiratory system were responsible for more visits to a doctor than those of any other system of the body. That is true because of the many problems in infants and children involving respiratory infections. In later years, beginning in the late twenties and thirties, and increasing with age, the digestive system goes to the top of the list.

This chapter will follow the same format as in the prior chapters, beginning with the anatomy and physiology of each part of the digestive system then going on to the most common disorders of that part of this very complicated apparatus. The discussion of pathology will follow immediately after the anatomy and physiology of each part of the digestive system.

THE MOUTH AND THE TEETH

The digestive system is basically a long continuous tube, beginning at the lips and ending at the anus. Along the way there are many solid structures that contribute to the digestive process and are essential to that process. We will start with the portal of entry; the mouth.

The lips serve a significant role in digestion. They keep the mouth closed while food is being chewed and swallowed. Their importance comes to our attention only if something happens to interfere with keeping the mouth closed, such as a severe injury to the lips or a neurological problem in which the nerve supply to the lips is damaged, preventing them from closing tightly. It is common to see drooling of food or saliva in older people who have had such a neurological event. Infections of the lips will be discussed in a subsequent chapter.

Immediately behind the lips are the teeth. They serve a very important role by chewing the food. Chewing reduces the size of the food particles and also mixes the food with the digestive enzymes of saliva.

SALIVA AND THE SALIVARY GLANDS

Saliva is taken for granted by most of us. It is common spit, a fluid that appears in the mouth when we chew. It is something to swallow or to expectorate with great flourish by tobacco chewers. In fact, however, saliva is a very complex fluid, containing very important digestive enzymes.

Enzymes are chemical compounds that are manufactured by the body in various organs to enable and facilitate chemical reactions within the body. Many enzymes serve important roles in the digestive process and many more serve in processes other than digestion. An earlier reference to enzymes was made in the discussion of the transfer of gases in and out of the blood within the lungs, facilitated by the enzyme carbonic anhydrase.

The enzymes in saliva are important in the digestion of carbohydrates. Actually, the process of digestion begins in the mouth with chewing, and continues through the esophagus, the stomach, and the intestines.

The enzymes found in saliva are produced by the salivary glands. They are two paired solid structures. The upper pair, called the parotid glands is located just in front and below each ear. They are about an inch to two inches in diameter and about one fourth of an inch thick. The saliva they produce flows through tubes called the parotid ducts and empties into the mouth through small openings located in the upper part of each cheek, just opposite the first molar tooth. For incidental intelligence only, that tube is called Stenson's duct.

The lower pair of salivary glands is called the submandibular glands. They are located in each side of the neck, just medial to the angle of the jaw. They are slightly larger than the parotid glands. The saliva they produce travels through a pair of ducts into the mouth, exiting at a fleshy projection on either side of the base of the tongue. Their ducts are called Wharton's ducts.

The outpouring of saliva from the salivary glands is controlled by the act of chewing, through a complicated set of nerves that go from the mouth into the brain. The sensory nerves tell the brain that eating has begun, or in some cases that eating is about to begin. The brain accepts the message and instantly tells the motor nerves to begin pouring out saliva. An interesting observation is that sometimes the nervous system gives the brain a premature signal that eating has begun. Have you ever noticed a spurt of saliva from the ducts under your tongue just as you are about to bite into a tasty hot dog? That was your digestive system just getting ready.

DISORDERS OF THE SALIVARY GLANDS

The most common of those is a stone (calculus) in a salivary gland or its duct. The stone is a solid lump, built up over time by crystallization of the minerals within the saliva. A small calculus can form within one of the salivary glands and be pushed into a duct by the flow of saliva. In most cases the calculus is small enough to pass through by itself, but if it is too large to pass it can block the duct completely. Then, as the gland produces more saliva, pressure builds up within the duct and backs up into the gland. The result is inflammation, with redness, swelling, pain, and local tenderness. The patient feels quite sick. In most cases a good head and neck specialist can remove the stone fairly easily. Occasionally the stone does not pass into the duct, but remains within the salivary gland until it is quite large. Often infection occurs, and the gland enlarges greatly. In some cases a major operation, requiring a skilled head and neck surgeon is necessary to remove a large calculus.

The next kind of problem affecting the salivary glands is infection. There are two kinds of infections seen here; viral and bacterial. A viral infection that has been largely eliminated by vaccination is mumps. In that disease a virus can invade all four salivary glands, or any combination of the four. The infected gland or glands become very swollen, tender and warm to touch on the overlying skin. There is complete recovery from mumps in most cases after two or more weeks of discomfort. It is wonderful to know that this disease has been virtually eliminated through routine immunizations.

Bacterial infections of the parotid salivary glands, called acute parotitis occur most commonly in the aged and in people who are severely weakened, or as a complication of surgery. The cause is thought to be, in most cases, severe drying of the mucus membranes of the mouth due to prolonged mouth breathing. That is the cause of most cases of acute parotitis, especially during sleep. Acute parotitis is a severe infection, requiring expert care. The treatment is usually the administration of antibiotics and medication to increase the flow of saliva. There is usually good recovery from this infection if proper treatment is given.

Tumors Of The Salivary Glands

The salivary glands are frequent sites of tumors. When they are benign they are called adenomas. If they are malignant they are called adenocarcinomas. They are usually discovered by the finding of a visible and palpable lump in one of the areas described above. When surgical consultation is obtained biopsies are usually taken of the tumor mass in an effort to determine whether the mass is benign or malignant.

Most often those tumors involve one of the parotid glands. The only proper treatment is surgical removal of the parotid gland if the tumor is malignant or removal of the tumor only if it is a benign growth. That surgery is best performed by a head and neck specialist because of the proximity of the important facial nerve to the parotid gland. With proper treatment most of those cancers can be cured. The absence of one parotid gland does not seriously affect digestive function.

We have now followed the pathway of food through the mouth, and have exposed the food to the first acts of digestion. Next the food enters the esophagus.

THE ESOPHAGUS

The esophagus is the beginning of the long tubular structure of the digestive tract. It extends from the back of the mouth downward through the chest (thorax), ending in the first part of the stomach. It has two layers, unlike most of the digestive tube. The innermost layer is a smooth thin sheet of cells called modified epithelium. Next is a thick layer of muscle arranged longitudinally. It is called the muscularis layer. The muscularis is the thickest component of the wall of the esophagus. The first portion of the muscular wall is composed of striated muscle that is under voluntary control. The remainder of the muscle of the esophagus is called smooth muscle that is not subject to voluntary control and receives its nerve supply from the autonomic nervous system, as do the muscles of the stomach, small intestine and large intestine. There is a discussion of striated and smooth muscle in the chapter on the musculoskeletal system.

In order to reach the stomach the esophagus passes through an opening in the diaphragm. The diaphragm is a thick, broad sheet of muscle that extends from front to back, and side to side, separating the thorax from the abdominal cavity with an airtight seal. It is that airtight quality of the diaphragm that permits the lungs to fill and empty with each breath.

The esophagus passes through an opening in the diaphragm that clings tightly against the esophagus, maintaining the airtight construction. That opening is called the esophageal hiatus of the diaphragm, leading to the gastro-esophageal junction.

DISORDERS OF THE ESOPHAGUS

In some people there is a weakness of the structures connecting the esophagus to the diaphragm. It is called a hernia. The full name then would be esophageal hiatal hernia. In severe cases of hiatal hernia much of the stomach is actually displaced into the thoracic cavity. In most cases of hiatal hernia however, there is merely a weak area at the G-E junction. That weakness permits reflux of the contents of the stomach backwards into the esophagus.

The esophagus, as the first true section of the digestive tube, has the duty of conducting and propelling digesting food through its lumen. That is done by means of the longitudinally arranged muscularis layer in its wall contracting in a sequential manner, pushing the contents down the tube. That function is carried out throughout the entire length of the digestive tract, propelling its contents toward the anus. That movement is called "peristalsis."

The esophagus is susceptible to a unique problem affecting the peristaltic muscle contraction. If we swallow something that is difficult to pass it sometimes sticks within the esophagus. That something in my own case is some sticky food, such as cottage cheese or peanut butter. In other people it may be very cold or hot liquid, or simply too big a swallow. When that occurs the lump of food, called a "bolus" of food in medical parlance, sticks within the esophagus. The esophagus then tries to expel the bolus by reversing the direction of the peristaltic wave. That causes a spasmodic contraction of the diaphragm. The antiperistaltic wave meets the peristaltic wave coming down the other way, and the diaphragm contracts repeatedly to expel the bolus. The result is a phenomenon that we all recognize as a hiccup.

Hiccups are usually a minor problem, cured by drinking some water, or other liquid. Sometimes they are very persistent, even requiring hospital care, but that is rare. I would like to offer my family recipe for overcoming persistent hiccups. Take a large glass of water. Stand up. Bend forward and drink the entire contents from the edge of the glass that is away from your body. In order to do that the water must travel uphill, which requires a strong peristaltic wave to propel it down the tube. When that strong wave meets the antiperistaltic wave it often forces the bolus of food downward into the stomach, and the hiccups end. Try it-it often works.

After the bolus passes through the gastro-esophageal junction it is in the stomach.

DISORDERS OF THE ESOPHAGUS RELATED TO THE STOMACH

The most frequent complaint related to the esophagus and the stomach is gastro-esophageal reflux disease, well known by the abbreviation GERD. It is due to the reflux, or backward flow of highly acid gastric juice through the cardia of the stomach and into the esophagus. The thick lining of the stomach protects it from irritation and inflammation by the strong acid that it manufactures. The esophagus has only the thin layer of epithelium. When the strong acid comes in contact with the esophageal lining it is severely irritating. The mucosa of the esophagus is supplied with sensory nerve endings that send a message to the brain saying 'heartburn'. The muscularis layer goes into spasm. The resultant discomfort is similar to the sensation of angina, but it also has a burning component, actually causing a sense of heat. GERD occurs mostly, but certainly not exclusively, in people who are overweight and eat too much at a single meal. Overfilling of the stomach causes a pressure sensation that is most easily relieved by escape of the gastric contents through the weak valve of the cardia. In people who are seriously overweight there is a buildup of fat within the peritoneal cavity that adds to the pressure on the stomach. The third component of reflux is the position of the patient. One should not lie down or sit in a deep chair for at least an hour after a large meal in order to minimize the likelihood of reflux.

The component of GERD that has received the most attention from the medical profession and from the pharmaceutical companies is the acidity of the stomach. Products for the reduction of stomach acid were the largest selling of all medications in the world in the year

2003. Those prescription medications are the greatest moneymakers for their manufacturers of any medicines in the world. In addition to prescribing those medications it should also be the role of physicians to educate their patients about the need to lose weight, to eat only foods that they know by experience their stomachs will tolerate, and to avoid those substances and foods that are on their personal no-no list, arrived at by their bitter experience. It is also important to remain vertical for an hour after meals. That common sense approach goes a long way toward minimizing the discomfort of GERD. It also empowers the patient to take charge of his or her own body.

The events of esophageal reflux and hiccups discussed above fall under the heading of recurrent acute esophagitis if they are only now and then episodes. If GERD occurs frequently and is an ongoing problem the inflammation of the esophagus then becomes classed as chronic esophagitis. Things can get quite serious then. When the lower inch or two of the esophagus remains chronically inflamed it can undergo a malignant change. The cells of the mucosa thicken and take on a different appearance from normal cells. That condition is called Barret's esophagitis, after the doctor who first described the change. If that condition is not relieved by treatment it can continue changing into a highly malignant form of cancer of the esophagus. Esophageal cancer is not rare. It requires extensive treatment and has a rather poor prognosis. It is very much worth the effort to avoid having chronic esophagitis by following the above precautions in order to avoid that major disease.

We have followed the digesting food through the esophagus and into the stomach. Now we come to that portion of the digestive tube that is truly within the abdomen. At this point we will take a break from our tour, and instead turn our attention to a very basic subject. In order to more easily understand the anatomy and workings of the digestive system it is a great advantage to have knowledge of the anatomy of the abdomen and of the peritoneal cavity. Those will be our next focus of study.

THE SURFACE ANATOMY OF THE ABDOMEN

In the discussion of the digestive system and in the chapters to follow we will deal with structures that are within the abdominal cavity and in the various regions of the abdomen. For the purpose of ready location of those structures it helps a lot to locate them in relation to the surface landmarks of the abdomen. This is the standard anatomic reference system that is used by all surgeons and practitioners of medicine.

The abdomen is bounded superiorly by the margins of the lowest ribs and inferiorly by the groins, (inguinal folds). In approximately the middle of the abdomen is the belly button, (umbilicus). The rear (posterior) boundaries of the abdomen are the muscular structures of the back. If a line is drawn across the lowest rib margins the space in the inverted V of the ribs is called the epigastrium. To either side of that space are the right upper quadrant and the left upper quadrant of the abdomen. The space on either side of the umbilicus is called the peri-umbilical region. On either side of that are the right and left mid-abdominal regions. Those extend to the right and left flanks, bounded inferiorly by the bony brim of the pelvis, and posteriorly by the muscles of the back. Below that level in the midline is the suprapubic region which extends to the pubic bone .On either side are the right and left lower quadrants of the abdomen. Remember these anatomical names. They will be used frequently in further discussions.

THE PERITONEAL CAVITY

The entire space within the abdomen is called the peritoneal cavity. Within that cavity are the stomach, the intestines, and the solid organs of the digestive system; the liver and the gall bladder. The pancreas, kidneys, adrenal glands and spleen are located behind the peritoneum, and are therefore called "retroperitoneal organs."

The reason for naming this cavity "the peritoneal cavity" is that the entire cavity is lined by a continuous sheet of serous (smooth and slippery) membrane called the peritoneum. That membrane is similar to the pleura that lines the thoracic cavity. The peritoneum has a rich blood supply and nerve supply. The peritoneal cavity is sterile; meaning that under normal conditions there is no bacterial life within its envelope. The digestive tube, on the other hand, has an enormous population of bacteria throughout its length. Those are essential to the digestive process. If a hole of any sort develops within the digestive tube there is liberation of bacteria and digestive juices into the peritoneal cavity. That causes severe Inflammation. When the peritoneum becomes inflamed that is called "peritonitis", bacterial or chemical or both. This occurs if a gastric ulcer perforates the stomach, spilling the highly irritating contents of acid and digestive enzymes into the peritoneal cavity. Peritonitis also occurs if any part of the intestine ruptures or becomes perforated.

In addition to the peritonitis caused by bacterial infection, there is chemical peritonitis. That is caused by the release of irritating substances from a diseased structure, such as the pancreas, which manufactures digestive enzymes and the gall bladder that stores bile.

Acute peritonitis can be diagnosed by the patient's symptoms, usually abdominal pain, nausea and vomiting, and the physical signs: progressive fever, tenderness and firmness and rigidity of the abdominal wall when presser, and reduction and then cessation of the motility and digestive sounds of the intestines. These will be discussed in detail in the following section on acute appendicitis.

ANATOMY AND PHYSIOLOGY OF THE STOMACH

The stomach is about twelve inches in length and six inches in diameter in the average adult. It is capable of extreme expansion when filled with food, and contracts when empty. It is transversely located in the upper abdomen, extending from left to right. The first portion of the stomach, the cardia, is the point of connection with the esophagus. That is called the cardio-esophageal junction. From there the stomach extends in a somewhat downward- sloping direction to the right mid-abdomen. The mid-section of the stomach is called the fundus, which terminates in the final section called the pylorus. There the stomach makes connection with the first portion of the small intestine, called the duodenum. The pyloric region ends in a muscular valve called the pyloric sphincter.

The wall of the stomach has four layers. The innermost layer is called the mucosa. It is very thick, with an intensely glandular lining. Within the mucosa are located the chief cells and the parietal cells that make strong hydrochloric acid and the enzymes that enable the digestion of protein. Just outside of the mucosal layer is the submucosa, containing nerves and blood vessels. Next is the muscularis layer composed of smooth muscle that contracts sequentially, churning the digesting food, and passing it along the digestive tube. The outer layer is called the serosa. That is a smooth, slippery membrane, enabling the peristaltic movements of the stomach within the peritoneal cavity. The internal environment of the stomach enables the digestion of those foodstuffs that are soluble in acid. At the pyloric valve the liquid digesting food leaves the stomach and enters the duodenum, which is the first portion of the small intestine.

GASTRIC (STOMACH) ULCERS

Most gastric ulcers are benign. The cause is chronic gastritis; (inflammation of the gastric mucosa). One cause of gastric ulcer formation is an infection by a bacterium called Helicobacter Pylorii, or H. Pylorii, in medical abbreviation. The means of contracting that infection is person-to-person, although the mechanism is unclear. H. Pylorii infection causes acute and chronic inflammation of the gastric mucosa, leading to high acid concentration and changes in motility of the stomach. H. Pylorii infection can be successfully treated with a regimen of antibiotic and antacid medication. Another underlying cause of gastric ulcer can also be emotional, the result of severe sustained stress, causing over-activity of the vagus nerve, which causes the gastric mucosa to hyper-secrete, and the gastric muscle activity to slow down. Reducing the acid production of the stomach, and increasing gastric motility with orally taken medications can usually successfully treat that kind of ulcer. Also to be considered is the patient's personal habits. Alcohol is a common cause of chronic gastritis. In some cases the choice of highly spiced foods can do the same thing. Of course, if the cause of chronic gastritis is severe emotional dysfunction the treatment becomes more complicated, but not less necessary. Psychotherapy is sometimes very helpful in such cases.

There is another cause of gastric ulcer that is much more sinister. That is cancer of the stomach. Virtually all gastric malignancies originate in the stomach, and are not metastatic from cancer elsewhere in the body. These are highly malignant cancers that have a high likelihood of metastasizing to other organs, chiefly the liver. The prognosis for gastric carcinoma is usually very poor.

ANATOMY AND PHYSIOLOGY OF THE SMALL INTESTINE

There are three sections to the small intestine; the duodenum, the jejunum, and the ileum. The duodenum is ten to twelve inches in length and the combined length of the jejunum and ileum is about twenty to forty feet, depending on the size of the adult individual. The construction is four layered, as in the stomach, but the anatomy of the mucosal layer is markedly different from that of the stomach.

The duodenum is the site of entry of two very important structures of the digestive system that lie outside of the food tube: the pancreas and the gall bladder. Those will be discussed in detail presently, but at this time it is their products that enter the duodenum that are of prime interest.

The pancreas manufactures two very powerful digestive enzymes called lipase and amylase that facilitate the digestion of fat and carbohydrate respectively. Those enzymes enter the duodenum via the pancreatic duct.

The gall bladder is the storage receptacle for bile, a strongly alkaline liquid that is manufactured in the liver, stored in the gall bladder and enters the duodenum via the bile duct, which merges with the pancreatic duct.

When digesting food is in the stomach specialized glands within the stomach release a hormone called cholecystokinin that is secreted into the blood stream. The presence of cholecystokinin stimulates the gall bladder to secrete bile into the bile duct, there to mix with the pancreatic enzymes, and to enter the duodenum.

The presence of bile and the pancreatic enzymes causes the internal environment of the duodenum to be one of very strong alkalinity, in contrast to the strongly acid environment within the immediately adjacent stomach. Each of those environments is uniquely suited to enable the digestion of different foodstuffs. Those environments are held separate by the powerful pyloric valve.

The mucosa and submucosa of the entire small intestine is adapted for the absorption of nutrient substances from the digesting food within its lumen. Oxygen and metabolites from the various organs of the body are supplied to the entire intestine by the arterial system.

The entire small intestine is free within the peritoneal cavity. It is suspended within a sheet of connective tissue called the mesentery. The entire blood supply of the small intestine, both arteries and veins, is carried within the mesentery.

The venous drainage of the mesentery throughout the intestine is very unique. Nutrients from within the lumen of the intestine drain into a very special system of veins called the portal vein system. The collecting veins from the entire intestine, carrying blood rich with nutrients from the intestinal lumen then drain into a major vein that is called the portal vein.

The portal vein then delivers that blood directly into the liver where major miracles of metabolism are done. The liver will be discussed in a following section.

In the previous chapter on the circulatory system there was a description of a severe intra-abdominal emergency event; a thrombosis of a mesenteric artery. That is a fairly common surgical emergency. The repair involves removing the devitalized segment of intestine and connecting the interrupted ends of viable intestine. That operation is usually quite successfully completed,

state called regional ileitis, which is synonymous with regional enteritis, or terminal ileitis, or Crohn's disease, depending upon whom you read. This is really a terrible disease. It is an acute and chronic inflammatory disorder. The current concept is that it is just another form of Crohn's disease, a very severe intestinal inflammatory disorder. These diseases are all classified as autoimmune disorders. The actual cause is not known. . In the case of regional ileitis there is severe inflammation of the mucosal lining. There is loss of the ability to function in the digestive process, severe diarrhea, often very bloody, severe pain, weight loss, anemia, and in some cases, death.

Regional Ileitis typifies Crohn's disease. It is quite different from other inflammatory conditions of the stomach or small intestine, such as acute gastritis or acute duodenitis. They are due to an entirely different cause, and are rarely as severe and crippling as acute regional ileitis.

This disease most often occurs in teenagers and young adults. The most successful treatment, often before and after surgery is suppression of the immune system with various medications. Corticosteroids and other anti-inflammatory drugs are commonly used for very long periods. In cases of severe scarring deformity of the ileum, or perforation, surgical removal of the affected segment is required.

INTESTINAL OBSTRUCTION

This is a common surgical emergency that can occur in people of any age. The small intestine, being quite mobile within the peritoneal cavity is particularly susceptible to this problem. The most frequent cause is the presence of adhesions within the peritoneal cavity. Adhesions are bands of tough, stringy tissue within the peritoneal cavity, formed as the result of previous peritonitis due to acute appendicitis or some other severe cause of inflammation. A loop of small intestine can become caught within bands of adhesions and not be dislodged. When that occurs, the segment of intestine that is trapped is usually in the form of a loop., With the passage of time the blood supply, both arterial and venous, becomes cut off. That is referred to as a closed loop intestinal obstruction. The intestine soon loses its vitality, and the process of gangrene occurs. The events of peritonitis follow, with the signs and symptoms described earlier. If a surgical operation is not performed soon the patient could likely die. At surgery the trapped intestine must be released. Quite often the intestine within the closed loop is found to be devitalized (dead), and must be removed. In most cases the surgeon can find the healthy ends of intestine and can re-establish the continuity of intestinal flow.

Hernias involving the muscular wall of the abdomen can at times entrap segments of intestine. In that case it is usually possible to release the involved intestine and repair the hernia before the intestine becomes devitalized, but that is not always possible, and in that case the dead segment must be removed.

We have covered the most common problems that involve the small intestine. Now let's go on to the large intestine.

THE LARGE INTESTINE, (THE COLON)

Names that are used synonymously are the colon, the bowel, and the large bowel. The entire intestine, beginning with the duodenum, and ending with the rectum is often referred to as "the gut" in serious medical parlance. For clarity we will use the term "colon" in discussing the large intestine.

ANATOMY AND PHYSIOLOGY OF THE COLON

The colon begins in the right lower quadrant of the abdomen, at the point where the ileum terminates. The first part of the colon is the greatest in diameter of any part of the intestine, from four to six inches. That portion is called the cecum. There is a valve at the junction of the ileum and the cecum, called the ileo-cecal valve. The ileum lies in a mainly transverse plane, and the cecum is in a vertical plane. The cecum extends cephalad for about four or five inches, after which the caliber of the colon narrows to about three or four inches. A very important fact to remember is that near the lowest portion of the cecum there is a narrow tube with a closed end that projects from the lumen of the cecum. That tube is the infamous appendix. We will return to the appendix in some detail.

Beginning with the cecum the vertical segment of the colon is called the ascending colon, traveling in a superior direction. From the outset of our tour the stomach and intestine have been located within the peritoneal cavity. After the cecum the colon dives behind the peritoneum, and becomes a retroperitoneal organ.

The ascending portion of the colon rises to the top of the peritoneal cavity where it takes a turn to the left, lying retroperitoneally behind the liver. Because the Greek name for liver is "hepar" that turn is called the hepatic flexure of the colon. Following the hepatic flexure that portion of the colon is called the transverse colon. Although the ascending colon is located retroperitoneally, the transverse portion and the remainder of the colon are located intra-peritoneally. The transverse colon proceeds leftward, to the region of the spleen. There it takes a turn downward. That bend is called the splenic flexure of the colon. The colon then proceeds downward, (in an inferior, or caudad direction), and is called the descending colon, to the lowest part of the peritoneal cavity. There it takes an s-shaped curve, at which point it is called the sigmoid portion of the colon, (from the Greek for letter S) which is about three feet in length. The sigmoid colon leads to the rectum, a straight tube of about ten to twelve inches in length. The rectum extends to the anus, which is the opening through which the digestive tube leaves the body and fecal waste is expelled.

The internal anatomy of the colon is quite different from that of the small intestine. Where the small intestine has largely the function of mixing, the digesting food with the digestive enzymes and absorbing the digesting nutrients, the colon has the main function of preparing the digesting food for excretion from the body. When the digesting food enters the colon it is mostly in a liquid form. When it leaves the body, in the normal state of health the waste is largely in a semi-solid state.

The mucosa that lines the colon is very different from that of the small intestine. Its cells are adapted for the absorption of fluid. There are also large mucus-forming glands that have the function of secreting mucus into the lumen for the purpose of lubrication.

There are times when the colon is inflamed by dietary irritants or by viral or bacterial infections or by severe anxiety and other emotional states. At those times there is often a great outpouring of mucus and fluid from the mucus-forming glands. That is the condition called diarrhea. Fluid and mineral losses from diarrhea can be extremely severe, requiring hospital care for the intravenous replacement of fluid and minerals, (called "electrolytes" in Doctor Speak). The opposite state, constipation, occurs when the body falls behind in its fluid intake, or when there is not enough soft bulk in the diet to absorb the fluid in the colon and make a soft enough stool to pass through the food tube in order to be excreted from the body. Constipation can be caused by medications that suppress intestinal motility. Narcotic pain medications often cause severe constipation.

We have finished the anatomic and physiologic tour of the colon. The presentation has been brief, but I hope, sufficient to provide a rough working knowledge. We will now go on to the disorders of the colon.

DISORDERS OF THE COLON

The first disorder, and possibly the one most familiar to the reader is acute appendicitis. It is not truly a disorder of the colon per se, but because of its close relationship to the cecum this seems the best place to present ACUTE APPENDICITIS. The appendix is a tubular structure that projects outward from the lumen of the cecum. Its tip is closed, making it a blind -ended pouch. The usual length is about three inches, although shorter or longer appendices are not uncommon. The usual diameter is about one fourth to one half inch. Its lining is much like that of the small intestine. The appendix has no known function. It appears to be a vestigial remnant from some earlier generation of mankind. The appendix is a normally found structure in all people.

Acute Appendicitis

The thing that distinguishes the appendix is its propensity to become seriously infected, requiring surgical removal, (appendectomy). This is how it happens. Because the appendix has a lumen that is continuous with the lumen of the cecum, all digesting foods that pass through the cecum have free access to the appendix. Remember that the appendix has a closed tip that makes it a pouch projecting from the cecum. In some people, with no known predisposition, a particle of digesting food or a dried particle of stool can enter the appendix and become lodged inside its lumen because it is too large to get out. When that happens the flow of material in and out of the appendix stops. As we know, the contents of the entire intestine include a large population of bacteria that under normal conditions help in the digestion of food and the nutrition of the body.

When blockage of the lumen of the appendix occurs, the part that is distal to the obstruction becomes a closed breeding ground for its bacterial contents. This causes inflammation of the mucosal lining of the appendix. That is followed by the outpouring of fluid into the closed end of the appendix. As the bacteria multiply the products of their metabolism begin to exert pressure on the wall of the appendix. That pressure is augmented by the inflow of white blood cells to combat the infection. There is the accumulation of pus, which is a combination of the bacterial metabolism and the defending white blood cells. The portion of the appendix that is distal to the obstruction becomes more and more distended. The wall of the appendix weakens. If no surgical intervention is done the appendix ruptures, releasing its contents of pus into the peritoneal cavity. The result is acute peritonitis. If no intervention is done there is a high likelihood that the patient will die.

Acute Appendicitis—The Signs And Symptoms

The first awareness of trouble after the appendix becomes obstructed is abdominal pain—a "stomach ache." That pain can be felt in any area of the abdomen. It is often high in the epigastrium, or mid-abdomen, but is most frequently felt in the right lower quadrant. Next there is often nausea and vomiting, but usually not diarrhea. The patient feels feverish and begins to complain of sore areas in the abdominal wall. Up to this point the complaints have been entirely noted by the patient, and are called symptoms. Now we enter the area of physical signs, rather than symptoms.

The earliest reliable sign is tenderness in the right lower quadrant. Tenderness is the sensation of pain noted by the patient upon external pressure on an affected area. That sign is enhanced by rebound tenderness in the same area. As the degree of inflammation of the appendix becomes more severe the peritoneum becomes progressively more inflamed and peritonitis involving the entire abdomen ensues.

The developing peritonitis causes the intestinal peristalsis to become slowed. The abdominal muscles become rigid to touch. If the appendix ruptures, releasing its contents of pus into the peritoneal cavity the peristaltic activity of the intestines stops completely, and the bowel sounds become silent. That is a very ominous sign.

How To Diagnose Acute Appendicitis

First, pay attention to the patient's complaints of "stomach ache", especially if they become increasingly severe. Vomiting is a strong clue that something bad is occurring. Next, you can in most cases locate the appendix this way: draw an imaginary line from the patient's umbilicus,(belly button) to the point of the right hip, which can be felt on the outside of the upper thigh with firm pressure in most people. Next, find the mid-point of that line. That point is called McBurney's point. In most people it overlies the appendix, although there are exceptions. Now, press hard downward at that point with the tips of your fingers held rigid. If the patient has acute appendicitis this should cause severe pain. Next, release the pressure abruptly. The pain should become much more severe. That maneuver is called eliciting rebound tenderness. That is one of the most reliable sign of acute appendicitis. Hopefully, the bowel sounds will still be active, but they may be becoming softer. Now, phone your doctor, or 911 immediately. The patient should be taken to a hospital immediately because you have diagnosed a possible life-threatening disorder and the patient night need an operation A.S.A.P.

Those are the signs and symptoms of acute appendicitis. They are also the signs and symptoms of acute peritonitis involving any intra-peritoneal organ. The location varies with the location of the organ within the peritoneal cavity.

We have just gone through a classic case of acute appendicitis. However, as in most events in life, things sometimes occur differently than in the "classic" manner. We should look at two possible alternate scenarios.

First, there is a common situation in which women who are within the age range of ovulation commonly have some pain at the time of ovulation. German doctors coined a term for that pain: "mittelschmerz", which means pain in the middle (of the month). In some cases the pain can be quite severe because of some bleeding that can occur from the surface of the ovary at the instant of ovulation. If the ovulation occurs from the right ovary the signs and symptoms can mimic very closely those of acute appendicitis because the right ovary is located very close to the appendix. Many operations have been performed in this instance, and quite correctly, because it is best NOT to overlook the possibility that it could be acute appendicitis and very little harm is most likely done by a quick look.

The other exception to the classic case is that of an unusual location of the appendix, such as completely behind the cecum, placing the appendix retroperitoneally, (outside of the peritoneal cavity). That can mask the classic symptoms and signs and make the diagnosis very difficult. My best advice is that if it looks like acute appendicitis the patient should be hospitalized and examined by a surgeon A.S.A.P.

DISORDERS OF THE COLON (CONTINUED)

Returning to the subject of disorders of the colon, let's go on with a condition that is very similar to that of appendicitis. The appendix is a blind-ended tubular projection from the lumen of the cecum. Such a structure is properly named "a diverticulum" of the colon. In the case of the appendix the reasons it causes such trouble is that it has a narrow lumen in relation to its length, and that it is located at the very beginning of the colon, at which point the digesting food is largely liquid with some solid particles which may enter the lumen of the appendix and become lodged there.

Another kind of diverticulum is quite common in the colon of most people. Most of us have multiple small diverticuli scattered throughout our colons. They are not present at the time of birth, but develop because of repeated minor inflammations of the colon. The presence of diverticuli of the colon is called "diverticulosis." Diverticuli usually have quite a wide mouth and lumen and are quite short. Such diverticuli are rarely obstructed but they can become inflamed and at times infected. Such a process is called acute diverticulitis. The signs and symptoms are similar to those of acute appendicitis but rarely as severe. The signs of peritoneal inflammation can sometimes be present. Medical treatment is usually necessary, sometimes requiring hospitalization for close observation and intravenous antibiotic medication. Surgical treatment is rarely necessary.

Another disorder of the colon that can become a very serious illness is acute colitis. In many cases the disease is truly acute in that it can occur for a variety of causes and subside, never to return. There is a truly chronic form of colitis, called variously inflammatory bowel disease, or Crohn's disease, and is extremely destructive. That condition is similar to regional ileitis, which was described earlier, in that it is classed as an auto-immune disease. It can be a chronic disease state that begins early in life and lasts a lifetime. It can be fairly mild, and intermittent, or it can also be a raging fire in the colon, sometimes causing bleeding ulcers of the mucosa with much loss of blood in liquid stools. It also quite commonly causes such severe dysfunction and scarring that extensive surgical removal of the affected colon is necessary. As in many severe chronic disorders chronic colitis can be a fatal condition.

Colon Cancer

The colon is one of the most frequently seen sites of primary cancer. As in the case of all other cancers, the cause is not really known. Many theories have been advanced, but no definitive causes have been found. Colon cancer has a tendency to metastasize, especially to the liver. In its metastatic state it is often an incurable condition, leading to death. However, colon cancer can often be cured, if diagnosed before it metastasizes, by surgical removal of the involved segment of colon. For that reason early detection is strongly advised. Colon cancer is most often seen in people in their forties or older. Diagnosis can be enhanced by having regular physical examinations, including digital examination (with the doctor's finger in the patient's rectum) and stool examinations for microscopic traces of blood, because most colon cancers bleed slightly. After the age of forty an examination of the rectum and sigmoid colon should be performed every three years in asymptomatic men and women. If abnormalities are found a complete colonoscopy should be done. After the age of fifty, routine colonoscopy for men and women every three to five years is strongly advised. If colon cancer is detected too late (after it has metastasized) the prospects for cure are poor. Remember, there are no typical symptoms or signs of colon cancer in its early stage. It is a potentially curable disease if detected early enough.

Irritable Bowel Syndrome

There is one more very common disorder of the colon that deserves mention. It is called irritable colon, or irritable bowel syndrome, or spastic colon. It is manifested by abdominal discomfort, bloating, diarrhea or constipation, or alternating diarrhea and constipation, urgency to stool, usually immediately after eating, and loud bowel sounds, gurgling or roaring, easily heard by others, usually at inopportune times. The causes can be varied, such as food intolerances or heightened nervous tone of the bowel due to emotional states. If you are having those symptoms it is a very good idea to consult your doctor because good treatment is available. There is no known causative relationship between irritable colon and inflammatory bowel disease, or bowel cancer.

THE RECTUM

This is the final or terminal segment of the digestive tube. The name, in Greek, means "straight place", and that is descriptive, as the rectum is a straight tube that follows the s-shaped sigmoid portion of the colon. In most adults it is about twelve inches in length. The construction is similar to that of the descending and sigmoid portions of the colon except that it has only three layers, lacking a serosal layer. The rectum ends in the anus, the final outlet of stool. Volumes have been written about the rectum and its disorders but for our purposes I will describe only the most common of those.

By far the most common disorder is hemorrhoids. As in all other parts of the digestive tube there is a profuse vascular bed of arteries and veins in the submucosal layer. The veins in the rectal area are subject to swelling because of the need to sit on a toilet seat and to exert pressure in order to assist the passage of stool out of the body. The thin-walled veins in the submucosal layer of the rectum become stretched out, and press the thin rectal mucosa inward toward the lumen. That condition is called hemorrhoids. Because of the thin mucosal wall hemorrhoids have a tendency to rupture and to bleed into the rectal lumen. This results in bloody stools. Hemorrhoids and other problems of the rectum and the anus are most often treated by a surgical specialist. The earlier name of that specialty was Proctologist. That terminology has been changed to Colo-Rectal Surgeon. Most hemorrhoid problems are treated in the doctor's office, with good results. Very severe cases require hospital-type surgery.

Another very common problem with hemorrhoids is that the veins can become injured, at times from sitting on a hard seat, likely because of venous stasis from the pressure of prolonged sitting. The blood within the vein forms a clot, (thrombus). That condition is called a thrombosed hemorrhoid. It is usually painful, requiring medical care. In most cases thrombosed hemorrhoid can be successfully treated in the doctor's office.

The rectum is subject to the same problems as occur in most of the colon. Among the most severe of those is inflammatory bowel disease, causing ulcer-ation, bleeding and pain. That condition requires skilled medical care.

Another problem, seen largely in the gay community, is injury and infection of the rectum due to anal intercourse. As in heterosexual intercourse, unprotected sex is a common cause of transmission of all sexually transmitted diseases, especially HIV disease. Unfortunately, some of those diseases may be known to the donor before the exposure occurs and can lead to life-threatening disease in the recipient. The most notorious and unfortunately the most common of those is infection by the HIV virus, leading to the terrible disease known as

AIDS.

HIV infection is preventable. All it takes is the common knowledge of how it is communicated, and the common sense to use that knowledge. Casual sexual intercourse, whether it is homosexual or heterosexual is risky in today's climate. There are people out there who have HIV disease and do not know it, and there are those who know it and do not care enough to advise their sexual partners. The first are ignorant, and the second are frankly evil. Either of those is an unacceptable sexual partner, but cannot be avoided in the setting of casual sex, especially of the "bath house" variety.

For a long time after the first explosion of HIV disease the gay community became a lot more cautious about casual sex. That attitude has, very sadly, become reversed recently because of the mythical "cure" of HIV disease by modern drug therapy. It is simply untrue that there is a cure for HIV disease. The treatment is very expensive, and the progress of the disease is hideous to the time of the patient's demise.

The only successful treatment is to prevent exposure to the HIV virus. To do that requires a better choice of partners, however possible, and at the least, barrier protection with condoms. Anal penetration is terribly risky with strangers. The incidence of non-HIV infections from anal sex is quite high, especially with strangers.

Rectal Cancer

Cancer of the rectum is a common disease. The cause, as in all other cancers, is not known. It has the same life-threatening potential as any cancer of the digestive tract. The first evidence of its presence is usually bleeding from the anus with the passage of stool. That bleeding is usually painless. At any sign of bleeding from the rectum, (or of any unexpected bleeding from any site), medical attention should be sought. Rectal cancer can metastasize, so it is very important to get medical help before that can occur, if possible. Early surgical removal can cure the cancer in many cases.

THE ANUS

The anus is the junction of the inner world of the digestive tract and the great out of doors. The mucosa of the rectum undergoes a physical change at the anus, blending gradually from smooth, thin membrane into the skin of the surrounding area. The anal muscle is located about one half inch within the anal opening. It is circumferential, exerting a tightening effect when contracted, and loosening when relaxed. That muscle is called the anal sphincter. Its function is to retain the contents of the rectum until it is relaxed. The anal sphincter is under voluntary control, as opposed to the musculature of the entire digestive tract from the esophagus to the anus. It is most likely that every reader of this book has had the experience of squeezing that muscle to hold in the passage of stool at inopportune moments, then enjoying the passage of a B.M.when the muscle is relaxed.

Disorders of the Anus

Anal disorders are frequently related to the presence of hemorrhoids that are located close to the anus. The symptoms include bleeding and painful thrombosis, usually caused by sitting on a hard surface, or a bumpy hard surface that injures the anal region. That causes the blood in the regional subsurface veins to clot. Thrombosed external hemorrhoids present as bluish-to black swellings at the edge of the anus. They are painful and tender to touch. If left untreated most will gradually subside after about two weeks from the time of their appearance. Treatment rendered by any trained physician usually consists of injecting a local anesthetic, then opening the vein and expressing (squeezing out) the thrombus. The pain stops immediately and the incision usually heals very quickly, (in most cases). That procedure, in most cases can be done in a doctor's office.

Another painful condition is Anal fistula, called "fistula-in-ano" in Doctor Speak. It is a serious problem, and fairly common. It begins with an irritation in a pocket in the side of the anus, called a crypt. An infection in an anal crypt can form an abscess, which is a closed-in infection, not open to external drainage. The abscess extends through the anal mucosa and submucosal tissue, and finds its way to the skin where it presents as a swelling or as a hole draining pus. It is painful, red, and swollen. The only successful treatment is an operation in which the entire passage of the draining tract from the anal mucosa to the skin is opened surgically, cleaned out, and left to heal by itself to prevent re-forming of the abscess.

THE LIVER ("HEPAR")—ANATOMY AND PHYSIOLOGY

This is a large organ, consisting of a solid mass of cells, richly supplied with blood vessels. The liver is situated in the right upper quadrant of the abdomen, just under the diaphragm. In the average adult male it can be twelve inches in transverse diameter, about the same in longitudinal diameter and eight to ten inches thick. The blood supply is from the hepatic artery, the portal vein, and the hepatic vein. The hepatic artery provides oxygenated blood and metabolites from many organs of the body. The portal vein brings a direct supply of nutrients from the small intestine into the vast chemical factory of the liver, ending in the maze of tiny vessels that supply each cell. The hepatic vein system returns the blood from the liver to the inferior vena cava. That blood is then returned to the heart, and is distributed to every part of the body.

The liver is surely one of the most remarkably complicated organs in the body, possibly rivaling the brain in its complexity. It is a chemical factory composed of millions of cells, each of which has been shown to perform thousands of chemical reactions instantaneously. Nutrients from the digestive tube are acted upon by the enzymes within the liver cells and transformed into the chemical components of all the cells of our bodies and the source of energy to run the body. The liver cells detoxify toxic substances that might injure the body. Waste chemicals are excreted by its cells.

Old blood cells that have outlived their life span are destroyed by the liver cells and their components are transformed into bile which is essential for the digestion of fatty substances in the intestine. Running throughout the liver is a system of channels called bile canaliculi. They carry the bile into the bile ducts, the tubes that drain the bile into the gall bladder.

DISORDERS OF THE LIVER

Alcoholic Cirrhosis

The liver, while being an amazing chemical factory is very sensitive to poisoning by toxic substances. The most common of those is alcohol. Even a small amount of alcohol causes some minor liver damage, but the liver has the ability to recover from minor damage. The regular ingestion of large quantities of alcohol causes severe poisoning of the liver, resulting in a disease called cirrhosis of the liver. Death from alcoholic cirrhosis is very common worldwide. The liver can also be seriously damaged by the chronic inhalation of solvents and the ingestion of other toxic substances.

The symptoms and signs of cirrhosis of the liver, or of any acute inflammation of the liver; usually begin with jaundice, a yellowing of the skin and of the sclerae (whites) of the eyes, due to release of bile from the damaged liver cells directly into the blood stream instead of into the bile canaliculi. There is enlargement and tenderness of the liver, indigestion, weight loss, and malaise.

As the cirrhosis continues there is loss of muscle tissue tone and wasting of the body. The cirrhotic liver weeps blood plasma into the abdominal cavity because of damage to the liver cells. The plasma is rich in protein, which is therefore lost to the body as a source of nutrition. A form of starvation actually occurs, abetted by the fact that most severe alcoholics would rather drink than eat. As the damage to the liver cells progresses the cells are replaced by scar tissue and shrinkage of the liver into a hard lump of scar tissue follows, ending in death of the patient.

Viral Hepatitis

Severe viral infection of the liver, called viral hepatitis is a common disease. There are three main types, called hepatitis A, B, and C. Hepatitis A is passed from person- to- person by means of ingesting the virus. That most often occurs through eating foods that have been handled by an infected individual whose hands were not properly washed after a bowel movement. The living virus is excreted in the stool. Restaurants and fruits purchased from street vendors are the most likely sources. This occurs most often in under-developed countries, but the carrier can be someone living in a modern city, who does not wash his or her hands. In most cases hepatitis A runs its course and the patient recovers in a few months, usually with no significant after-effects.

Hepatitis B and C viruses are carried in the blood of the infected person, and are passed from person-to-person by means of some kind of contact involving interchange of the donor's blood or other body fluid with that of the recipient. The most common contact is by means of hypodermic needles, chiefly in the case of drug addicts using old needles. Unprotected sexual intercourse is another common way of passing Hepatitis B or C because of the exchange of bodily fluids through abrasion of the mucous membranes of the recipient's vagina or rectum. Both hepatitis B and C are passed in those ways. Both are lifelong infections for which there is no known cure. It is quite common for people to die from hepatitis B or C infections that either acutely or chronically destroy the cells of the liver. Hepatitis C has been implicated as a cause of primary cancer of the liver.

The earliest signs of all types of viral hepatitis are fever and jaundice, severe weakness and malaise. It causes the patient to be generally very sick. In most cases the disease does not destroy the liver to the extent of severe alcoholic cirrhosis, but it can result in permanent liver damage, requiring liver transplantation to enable the patient to continue living. Both hepatitis B and C are common causes of death. Liver transplantation is often quite successful if the problems of organ rejection can be overcome. That option is usually not available in the case of alcoholic cirrhosis because most of the body tissues are so damaged by alcohol that a new liver would be of no avail.

Cancer Of The Liver

Cancer of the liver is a very common disease. Most liver cancers are metastatic, having originated in other organs of the body and been carried to the liver by the blood stream. Within the liver the cancer cells usually grow rapidly. That disease has a very poor prognosis.

There are some primary cancers of the liver that originate in that organ. They are much less common than the metastatic cancers. Some primary liver cancers can be cured completely by surgical removal of the cancerous area.

The symptoms and signs of liver cancer vary with their location within the substance of the liver. As a general rule there is fatigue, malaise and loss of appetite with conspicuously rapid weight loss. There is usually progressive jaundice caused by the liberation of bile from damaged cells. The liver may be enlarged and palpable early in the disease. That becomes more evident as the disease progresses. Weakness and severe weight loss are very evident late in the course of the disease, along with enlargement of the abdomen due to the increased size of the liver and the accumulation of intra-abdominal fluid.

Liver Function Tests

There are a number of blood tests that are used to measure the functioning of the liver. They are based on the fact that the liver produces enzymes that are vital for the processes of digestion and metabolism of nutrients. In good health those enzymes remain largely within the cells of the liver. Levels of those enzymes can be measured by specific blood tests. In conditions in which the liver cells are damaged those enzymes are liberated into the blood stream in greater quantities and can be measured accurately. Liver enzyme tests are used to track the progress of cirrhosis, viral infections and cancer of the liver, and are very useful in determining the status and prognosis of the disease.

THE GALL BLADDER

As bile is manufactured by the liver cells from the recycled contents of old red blood cells it is collected by the tiny bile canaliculi and transported to the hepatic duct and the common bile duct which carry the bile into the gall bladder.

The gall bladder is a pear-shaped sac that is suspended below the liver. Its size is variable, but in the average adult it is about four to six inches in length, and three to five inches in diameter when filled with bile. When bile enters the gall bladder it's a thin golden-colored liquid. It is stored there until required for assistance in digesting a fatty meal. During storage in the gall bladder some of the water is absorbed from it, and it thickens and assumes a greenish color.

When fatty digesting food leaves the stomach a hormonal substance, called cholecystokinin is produced and released into the blood stream. Cholecystokinin is carried to the gall bladder and stimulates it to contract, squeezing out bile. The bile flows through a tube called the cystic duct into the common bile duct, then into the lumen of the duodenum. There the bile mixes with the digestive enzymes produced by the pancreas and encounters the digesting fatty food. Acting as a detergent in the kitchen sink, bile breaks the water/fat barrier that surrounds the food. That permits the digestive enzyme, lipase, to break the digesting food into its chemical components. In that form the nutrients are absorbed through the mucosa of the intestine and carried by the portal vein into the liver.

DISORDERS OF THE GALL BLADDER

The most frequent disorder of the gall bladder is the development of gall stones. That name is given to solid masses that form within the gall bladder, beginning as crystals that precipitate out of the stored bile. Most gall stones are composed of cholesterol, calcium and lecithin, a solid polymerized fat. Stones occur quite commonly in women in their forties who have had one or more pregnancies. That is thought to be because as the enlarging uterus presses upward in the abdomen it causes compression of the bile ducts and the gall bladder. That slows the egress of bile, allowing the bile to remain in the gall bladder longer than usual. When the bile stands still for too long within the gall bladder crystal form with subsequent layering that results in gallstone formation. There are also hormonal factors in pregnancy that further enable the formation of gall stones. Of course, men also have gall stones, but less frequently than do women, not due to the same conditions, but probably due to the same mechanism of gradual layering.

One problem that occurs with gall stones is that small stones can slip down, out of the large space of the gall bladder and into the common bile duct. In most cases the stone will pass through the narrow space of that passage into the duodenum and will be excreted with the stool.

However, it is often the case that the stone is too large to pass and becomes lodged in the common bile duct. That results in complete blockage of the outflow of bile. The patient immediately experiences severe pain in the right upper quadrant of the abdomen, often accompanied by nausea and vomiting. There is often jaundice, due to the backing-up of bile into the liver and from there into the venous system. As the obstruction goes on the patient can develop signs of peritonitis. If surgical intervention is not done the gall bladder can rupture, causing the release of bile into the peritoneal cavity. That causes chemical peritonitis and ultimately, death of the patient if prompt surgical treatment is not done. At the time of onset of any of the above symptoms the patient becomes incapacitated. A surgical emergency has occurred. A surgeon should see the patient as soon as possible.

As a general rule, most surgeons would hospitalize the patient for treatment of pain and for observation. With any luck the stone will pass, symptoms will abate, and the acute inflammation will subside. Then, in a week or two, the patient should have the gall bladder removed because it is diseased. Only in very rare cases are the stones removed, leaving the gall bladder intact.

If the symptoms and signs worsen, the surgeon may be forced to operate under emergency conditions. That increases the risks and hazard of the surgery greatly.

With modern surgical technique the preferred type of operation is with the use of the Laparoscope. With that instrument a tiny television camera is inserted into the abdomen through a small incision. Two or three other similar incisions are made for the introduction of small surgical instruments. The surgeon views the interior of the abdomen on a closed circuit television screen and with the small instruments dissects the gall bladder free of its attachments and removes it.

In the case of a need for emergency surgery the contents of the abdomen may be too inflamed and fragile to permit laparoscopic surgery with safety. In that case the older technique of making a long incision in the right upper quadrant of the abdomen and the removal of the gall bladder under direct vision is the safer procedure, although the healing and recovery times after surgery are much longer.

Cancer of the gall bladder is very rare, but does occur. The signs and symptoms are those of gradual obstruction of the outflow of bile, usually with jaundice, and indigestion, weight loss, weakness, and malaise. The treatment depends upon the nature of the disease process that is present.

THE PANCREAS

The pancreas is another major digestive organ that is located within the abdomen but outside of the digestive tube. It's a solid organ, located retro-peritoneally, approximately posterior to the gastro-duodenal junction, or behind the umbilicus. Its average size is about six inches in transverse length by four inches in longitudinal measurement, and two or three inches in antero-posterior thickness.

The pancreas has two widely disparate types of cells that perform completely different functions. The major bulk of the organ is a digestive gland that manufactures two very important enzymes; lipase, which is essential for the digestion of fatty food and diastase, which assists in the digestion of carbohydrates. Those are secreted into the duodenum through the pancreatic duct which is joined by the common bile duct just before the point of entry into the duodenum.

The other function of the pancreas is due to clusters of cells called The Islets Of Langerhans. Those cells produce the hormone insulin. The islet cells, also called beta cells are in a close relationship with veins that receive the insulin and carry it, via the vena cava, to the heart where it enters the arterial circulation and is delivered to all parts of the body. A normal supply of insulin is essential for the metabolism of sugar. If a deficiency of insulin occurs the individual becomes diabetic. Conversely, insulin is the standard medication for the treatment of a form of diabetes. Diabetes will be covered in detail in the chapter on the endocrine glands.

Two main types of severe disorders can affect the pancreas. One is acute pancreatitis, which is an inflammation of that organ. The cause of acute pancreatitis is not known, but there may be some causal relationship with inflammatory disorder of the stomach which lies adjacent to the pancreas. Severe gastritis, frequently due to alcohol excess, can be followed by an attack of acute pancreatitis.

When the pancreas becomes inflamed its digestive enzymes attack the cells of the pancreas itself, causing their breakdown. That releases more digestive enzymes that then attack the adjacent tissues within the peritoneal cavity. The result is much like a severe forest fire. The entire peritoneal cavity becomes inflamed. Acute peritonitis occurs. The bowel becomes paralyzed, and bowel sounds cease. The pain is said to be the most severe that anyone can experience, requiring heavy narcotic medication for relief. There is very little in the way of active therapy to offer a person with acute pancreatitis. No food or liquid is allowed in order to minimize stimulation of the pancreas. Heavy sedation and analgesic medication is given, and some medications to reduce the inflammation may be effective. No surgical remedy is possible. The patient must lie in a hospital bed awaiting recovery. Death from severe acute pancreatitis is not uncommon.

Cancer of the Pancreas

The other severe disorder of the pancreas is cancer. Primary cancer of the pancreas is not an uncommon disease. Because of the location of that organ the cancer causes severe damage to the very sensitive adjacent structures. Surgery for pancreatic cancer is in its infancy and is very hazardous. Alternative medical therapy is rarely successful. There is a very high mortality rate from this disease.

Chapter Four
THE URINARY SYSTEM

This part of the body is the "water works." It consists of the kidneys, the ureters, the bladder, and the urethra in both sexes. The prostate, in men, is rightly a part of the reproductive system but is usually treated by urologists and therefore is included in this chapter.

All living organisms require water in order to exist, with the possible exception of some viruses. Humans take in water from the digestive tract. Water is a by-product of the metabolism of most tissues. The ingested water and the waste water are brought to the urinary system via the blood stream. In the urinary system the blood is filtered. The majority of the water is returned to the general circulation to be used by all tissues of the body. Within the urinary system waste products are filtered out in their water medium. The waste is excreted from the body as urine. A small but important amount of water is lost from the body from breathing, and in the form of sweat.

THE ANATOMY AND PHYSIOLOGY OF THE URINARY SYSTEM

The anatomic structures of the urinary system in most people consist of two kidneys, each located in the retroperitoneal space behind the lowest rib in the area called the flanks. There are two ureters, each connected to one kidney. Ureters are long tubular structures that conduct urine from the kidneys to the urinary bladder. The bladder is located in the midline in the area just above the pubic bones, at the bottom of the abdomen. That is referred to as the suprapubic region. The urine leaves the bladder through a tubular structure called the urethra which conducts it out of the body. We will now look at those structures in detail.

The kidneys are about the size of a man's fist. They are composed of a solid portion, called the renal cortex, ("ren" is the Greek word for kidney, hence references to the parts of the kidney that are called "renal"). The renal cortex consists of millions of small filtering cells, arranged in groups called glomeruli. It is within the cortical portion of the kidney that waste products, dissolved in the water that brought them, are filtered out of the blood through the glomeruli and the rest of the water is returned to the general circulation. An important part of the filtration apparatus through which all the urine passes is a series of long tubes called the renal tubules.

After the filtration process the waste water and its contents are passed on to the medullary portion of the kidney. In the medulla the newly formed urine is led into the collecting tubules and from there into the renal pelvis.

The renal pelvis is a capacious structure that conducts the urine into the ureters. Each ureter is a three-layered tube consisting of an inner layer called the endothelium which is thin, smooth and richly supplied with blood vessels and nerves. The middle layer, called the muscularis layer is composed of smooth muscle that is usually in a state of relaxation, but is capable of contraction, moving the flow of urine from the kidneys into the bladder. The ureters are capable of contracting, reducing the caliber of the lumen. The outside layer is a thin fibrous material called adventitia. The lumen of the average ureter is about one eighth to one fourth of an inch in diameter in its relaxed state. The length of a ureter varies with size of each person.

The ureters conduct the urine into the urinary bladder, which is commonly referred to as "the bladder." There is a point of narrowing of the ureteral lumen at its point of connection with the pelvis of the kidney and another at the point of connection with the bladder. The former is called the uretero-pelvic junction and the latter the uretero-vesical junction.

The bladder is a large bag-like structure that has a capacity of about one to two pints, depending on the individual. It has a three-layered wall, much like that of the ureters. The muscle layer is very thick and strong. The muscle wall of the bladder is smooth muscle, not subject to conscious effort, in the same manner as the muscle of the entire digestive tract. In its relaxed state it permits the maximal capacity of the bladder. When it contracts it can wring out the urine contents to a capacity of nearly zero, again depending on the individual.

The urethra has a much wider lumen than that of the ureters, usually at least one-fourth inch in diameter. The length of the urethra varies greatly with the individual. In women it extends from the bladder to a point just above the vaginal opening. That is about one and a half to two inches on the average. In men the urethra extends from the bladder opening through the penis, and so is highly variable in length.

There is a strong muscle at a point just beyond the bladder in both sexes. It is circumferential and so is called the urethral sphincter. That sphincter is composed of striated muscle and functions upon positive command of the individual.

In the normal individual when that muscle is contracted the passage of urine out from the bladder stops. When the urethral sphincter relaxes, and the muscle layer of the bladder contracts the urine flows out of the bladder.

DISORDERS OF THE URETHRA AND THE BLADDER

In most sexually active young adults problems involving the urethra and the bladder stem from sexual intercourse or pre-intercourse fondling. The suffix "-itis" is used to describe infections of the urinary organs, even though you and I know that it really means inflammation.

As in the case of the term "appendicitis" there is always severe inflammation associated with the infection. That is also the case in urinary tract infections.

Bladder infections are extremely common in young women and in women who are not experienced in sexual intercourse. For reasons that are obscure to me the tendency to have those infections subsides as women continue to be sexually active-in most cases. The best explanation is that the body's defenses are able to adapt to the new conditions imposed by being sexually active.

In women bladder infection (urethro-cystitis) usually occurs as the result of vaginal bacteria entering the urethra during sexual penetration or even with fondling of the genitals. One reason for this is that the entire urinary tract, from urethra to kidneys is sterile (having no bacterial population) in normal females. The vagina, however, has a large population of bacteria as a part of its normal flora. The female urethra is so short that it does not provide a barrier against the ingress of bacteria into the bladder. The introduction of bacteria which are normal and essential as flora of the vagina causes an infection of the urethra and bladder. Of course, there are also those infections caused by pathogens (organisms known to cause disease) such as the bacteria of gonorrhea, but those are much less commonly the culprits.

The symptoms of acute urethro-cystitis are burning pain upon urination, increased frequency of urination and cramping pain in the suprapubic region after voiding. There is almost always blood in the urine. There is rarely fever unless the infection has extended beyond the bladder into the ureters. Fortunately, most lower-urinary tract infections can be cured with oral antibiotic therapy.

Infection of the urethra in males is quite common. It is also usually the result of sexual intercourse. In the case of males the infection can be prevented by the use of condoms. This is especially true in the case of anal intercourse. The bacterial content of the rectum is very highly infectious if it enters the urethra.

Because the urethra is much longer in males than in females it is unusual for a urethral infection to progress to a bladder infection in males. Such an event is usually the result of ignoring early symptoms which include itching within the penis, burning pain in the penis upon urination and then the sign of a purulent, (pus) discharge from the urethra.

Again, in most cases urethral infections in males can be successfully treated with oral antibiotics, although in the case of infections caused by anal intercourse the bacteria have recently shown evidence of becoming resistant to most antibiotics that can be taken orally.

Bladder Cancer

Bladder cancer is not a rare disease and seems to have increased in frequency in recent years. It is a relatively silent disease, meaning that it causes few symptoms. Blood in the urine (hematuria) is usually the first sign of trouble, and at that point the cancer can be quite advanced.

Bladder cancer can sometimes be cured by fairly conservative treatment if detected early but it may require radical surgery to achieve a cure if the cancer is advanced.

If any evidence of blood is noted in the urine it is imperative that a medical consultation should be had as soon as possible in order to determine the cause. There are other, less ominous, causes of bloody urine, but it is essential that bladder cancer be diagnosed and treated in its most early and curable state. Early consultation with a urologist is imperative.

DISORDERS INVOLVING THE URETERS AND BLADDER

The problem that affects the ureters most frequently is shared with the pelvis of the kidney. That problem is the passage of kidney stones that form in a kidney pelvis then enter the ureter. Solid particles are formed within the renal pelvis in a manner similar to that of gallstones in the gall bladder. Crystals of the substances being excreted by the kidneys precipitate out of solution and lie in the spacious renal pelvis. Over time those particles can enlarge, forming solid particles of greater size. Those particles are referred to as "stones." The correct medical terminology is "urinary calculi." A single stone is a "urinary calculus." At some point and for reasons that are not clear, one of those stones will leave the spacious confines of the renal pelvis and enter the ureter that drains that kidney. If the particle is not too large it will pass through the ureteropelvic junction and be washed by the flow of urine down to the ureterovesical junction. If it is small enough to pass through that narrow opening it will enter the bladder and eventually be washed out through the urethra and out of the body without the host being aware of the entire process.

If, however, the stone has become too large It may wedge into one of three places: the uretero-pelvic junction, or if it passes that, the point where the ureter crosses over the bony brim of the pelvis, of the ureterovesical junction. Regardless of which of those three points it reaches, the symptoms are the same. There is sudden very severe pain in the affected flank and in that side of the abdomen. The patient thrashes about, trying to find a comfortable position to make the pain go away. There may be some nausea and vomiting because of the severity of the pain involving the autonomic nervous system. That is because the muscles of the ureter go into spasm, probably in an effort to expel the stone, and that causes the wall of the ureter to clamp down on the stone, stimulating the rich nerve bed within the ureter to deliver a strong pain message to the brain.

The clinical signs include bleeding into the urine as the stone scratches the lining of the ureter, lacerating its blood vessels. There is usually tenderness on the affected flank, and possible tenderness in the affected side of the abdomen.

When this event is recognized it is essential to get medical help A.S.A.P. Strong analgesic medication is required, either by vein or by intramuscular injection. Once the pain has been overcome by medication the patient often goes to sleep. In that relaxed state the stone will often pass spontaneously. In some cases the pain subsides, only to recur when the effect of the medication wears off, because the stone has not passed. In that case it may be necessary to keep the patient in the hospital for several days.

In the modern treatment of kidney stones when the patient enters the emergency room, or is admitted to a hospital the first stop is the radiology department. There, usually using X-Ray examination, or occasionally an ultrasound study, the location and size of the stone are determined. If the symptoms persist for a lengthy time that study is repeated to see if the stone has advanced. There is usually a waiting period of several days to allow the stone to pass into the bladder.

In the event that the pain ceases, but the stone has not passed out, the patient is usually discharged to home on that date. The expectation is that the stone will pass through urethra and out of the body without incident. That is because the caliber of the urethra is much greater than that of the ureters, permitting most stones to pass. The patient is usually given a filter to be used for every urination in the hope of capturing the stone. It can then be analyzed chemically to determine its composition. With that knowledge a diet, low in those elements can be recommended in the hope of preventing further stone formation.

In the event that the pain persists and the stone is shown radiologically to have made no progress, at some point the decision is made to remove the stone surgically. In most cases that can be done through the urethra with an instrument called the operating cystoscope. That is usually a minor operation and usually quite successful. The patient is usually discharged on the day following the surgery.

Quite often the initial radiologic examination will reveal the presence of multiple stones, either in the affected renal pelvis or also in the opposite one. If the stones are small there is usually no treatment given other than a change in diet. Sometimes the radiologic study shows the presence of huge calculi that fill most of either or both renal pelves. Some of those are referred to as "giant", or "staghorn" calculi, because of their appearance filling the pelvis and extending into the collecting passages from the medulla of the kidney. To remove that type of calculi requires the use of a very special type of instrument called a Lithotripter that uses powerful sound waves to shatter the calculi into small fragments. Following that the fragments can be removed piecemeal through the renal pelvis, or by washout techniques.

A related problem is the discovery by the radiologist of ureteral strictures; narrowing of one or both ureters. Those are usually of congenital origin, and can be treated with dilation through the cystoscope.

An uncommon condition is acute ureteritis, which is an infection of one or both ureters, usually due to backwash from a severe bladder infection. That condition can be treated with antibiotic medication, usually with good results.

DISORDERS OF THE KIDNEYS

The words "renal", and "nephron", derived from Greek are commonly used to name the kidney, and the single filtering unit of the kidney comprising a glomerulus and its tubules. Those words are used frequently in the details of renal function and dysfunction.

Probably the most common disorder of the kidney is infection that ascends from the bladder through the ureters, and reaches the pelvis of a kidney. That infection is called "pyelitis". If the infection extends into the solid material of the kidney it is called "pyelonephritis." That can be a very serious infection, requiring heavy antibiotic therapy.

Polycystic kidney is a congenital disorder in which one or both kidneys develop with large fluid-filled spaces between the glomerular structures of the cortex. It is quite common. The open spaces are given the name "cysts." This condition is usually asymptomatic, and in most cases does not cause any loss of renal function. It is usually discovered accidentally in a radiologic study done to locate urinary calculi. That condition usually does not require any treatment.

A more serious and common disorder of the kidneys is called nephrosclerosis. That name refers to severe atherosclerotic change in the arterial blood supply of the glomerular filtration system. It is almost always accompanied by severe generalized atherosclerosis throughout the body. Because there is such an enormous blood supply to the millions of glomeruli within the kidneys the entire body is seriously affected. The individual's blood pressure becomes seriously elevated, and the efficiency of the filtering system is reduced. That results in a buildup of nitrogenous waste materials and mineral within the body. The treatment of that disorder requires complicated medical care given by experienced specialists.

Another and most devastating renal disorder is acute glomerulonephritis. That condition is also called "nephritis" or, especially in children, "the nephrotic syndrome." The Greek word for the filtering apparatus of the kidney is "nephron", and for the individual filter the "glomerulus." If you add our old friend, "-itis" to that, and understand that this is a disorder of the glomerulus filters of the renal cortex; the word "glomerulonephritis" makes sense. This disease is another member of that very severe family of diseases called auto-immune diseases. As in all diseases in that family, the exact mechanism of cause is not known.

Acute glomerulonephritis causes the glomerular filters to become inflamed, deformed, scarred and ultimately to cease functioning. When that happens, the waste materials of the body that are normally excreted by the kidneys accumulate in the bloodstream, and in the body tissues.

That causes poisoning of most of the organs of the body with the waste products. That state is called "uremia."

The symptoms of that disease can be mild at first. There is retention of salt and water with swelling of the hands, feet and face, and the collection of free fluid within the peritoneal cavity with distention of the abdomen. There is usually headache, fatigue and gradual malaise that becomes worse rapidly. The blood pressure rises and blood tests reveal an increase in nitrogenous waste products.

The usual first line of treatment is to attempt to suppress the Inflammation of the kidneys with corticosteroids and other immune-suppressant medications. If that is successful and the symptoms subside the patient is usually kept on those medications for a period of months to years in the hope that the inflammation will go away.

If that treatment is not successful and the waste products continue to rise in the blood stream, some effort is made to replace the filtering system of the kidneys with some type of external artificial filter. Dialysis in some form is started. That is done in two ways: Peritoneal dialysis in which tubes are inserted into the peritoneal cavity and the fluid is withdrawn and substituted with fluid that is free of waste products. That usually must be repeated at least once each week, often more frequently. For that reason the tubes are put in place surgically.

If peritoneal dialysis becomes inadequate to clear the waste products an artificial kidney can be employed. An artery and a vein are prepared as shunts that can be used repeatedly. They are then connected to a complex machine that filters the blood and returns it to the body. That technique is called renal dialysis. That usually has to be repeated once weekly, or more often. That treatment can be continued for years.

In the event that the artificial kidney becomes inadequate or if the frequency with which it is used becomes excessive, another kind of treatment can be used. One of the patient's diseased kidneys can be replaced with a healthy kidney from a donor. That is a very complicated process requiring finding a tissue match between donor and recipient to prevent rejection of the new kidney by the recipient's immune system. There may be a need for ongoing medication to prevent rejection, but that is the ultimate way to keep the patient alive following that terrible disease.

The management of this kind of "end-stage" disease of the kidney is most often done by physicians in the specialty of "Nephrology." Much research continues to be done in the field of Nephrology. New and better medications to treat the inflammatory diseases of the kidney have been developed. Cadaver renal transplantation, using donated kidneys from people who have assigned their body tissues for donation after their death, in addition to live donors, are now being used. This has greatly improved the prospects for survival for people whose kidneys have failed.

Cancer of the Kidney

There is one more disorder of the kidneys that must be discussed. That is the ever-present condition of cancer. Primary cancer of the kidney is not common, but does occur. The most common early symptom is the presence of blood in the urine. There can be pain in the affected kidney region, depending on the location and size of the cancer. Treatment depends on the nature of the cancer. Surgical removal of the affected kidney is usually done, followed by some type of specific therapy, again depending on the extent of the cancer. The outcome, again, depends on the specifics of the cancer.

Metastatic cancer reaching the kidney is a very uncommon condition. In the event of that occurrence treatment must be directed to both the kidney and to the primary organ of origin of the cancer.

Our tour of the urinary system has taken us through all of the parts that are common to both sexes. There is one more organ to discuss; the prostate.

THE PROSTATE

This organ is present in males only. It is a firm, solid structure, located at the base of the penis at the point where the urethra connects with the bladder. In most adult males it is about the size of a golf ball. It has three lobes, one on each side of the urethra, and a smaller median lobe.

It is composed mainly of fibrous tissue, but contains glands that make a fluid called semen. The semen is secreted into sacs called seminal vesicles where it is stored, then passed into the urethra at the time of ejaculation, and serves as a vehicle for the sperm cells.

DISORDERS OF THE PROSTATE

Prostatic disorders are rare in children. Problems are first seen in young adult males who are sexually active. They are chiefly infections. Infections of the urethra can ascend to the level of the prostate and cause acute prostatitis. That infection is usually signaled by pain and swelling and tenderness in the perineal region and a discharge from the urethra. Prostatitis can usually be treated successfully with oral antibiotic therapy.

In older males, usually beginning at about age fifty, prostate problems tend to become chronic, rather than acute. That means that the causes of the disorders may not readily be curable, as they are in the case of acute prostatitis.

By far the most common prostate problem that afflicts older men is ongoing enlargement of the prostate. That is called benign prostatic hyperplasia, or BPH.

Because the mass of the prostate surrounds the urethra at the outlet of the bladder the enlargement tends to act as a valve, narrowing the passage and slowing the outflow of urine from the bladder. That causes the stream of urine to be progressively weaker and slower, and the need to void more frequently, with smaller volumes of urine outflow each time. There is hesitancy in emptying the bladder and dribbling at the termination of voiding. That leads to inability to empty the bladder completely upon urination. As the prostate grows larger the volume of urine retained in the bladder after voiding grows larger. Thus, the man feels that he has emptied his bladder, but he may have retained as much as a quart or more of urine in his bladder.

That becomes a serious problem at bedtime. If a man goes to sleep with his bladder half full of urine it does not take long for the additional flow of urine from the kidneys to distend his bladder to the point of discomfort. That awakens him and he goes back to the bathroom only to have the same thing awaken him again. The number of nocturnal awakenings to void can reach six or eight, disturbing his sleep greatly. In some cases, because the bladder becomes so distended that it has no squeezing power to oppose the restriction of outflow, urinary retention occurs, and there is complete inability to pass urine.

At that point or possibly sooner the patient seeks medical help. He should be tested to rule out the possibility of cancer of the prostate. A rectal examination by a trained physician can reveal the presence of a mass within the prostate, which would be a clue to possible cancer. A blood test, called the Prostate Specific Antigen, or P.S.A., for short, can give a strong suggestion of the presence of cancer. Finally, needle biopsies of the prostate, a relatively painless procedure in most cases, can give microscopic evidence of the presence or absence of prostatic cancer. With cancer ruled out, the diagnosis is benign prostatic hyperplasia (B.P.H.) If the number of awakenings is three or four he may be advised to try a prescription medication. If that helps and if he can tolerate the number of awakenings that treatment may suffice. However, if the number of awakenings increases it is time to have some sort of surgical procedure.

In the past few years there have been a significant number of new surgical treatments offered, but in most cases the standard surgical technique is called Trans-Urethral Resection of the Prostate (T.U.R.P.). That is done through the penis with an electrical instrument that burns the tissue away and minimizes bleeding. Over the years that has remained the procedure of choice in the hands of most good urologists. The results are usually very satisfactory. In some cases in which the prostate is too large to permit satisfactory results with the T.U.R.P. The prostate is removed surgically through an incision.

Cancer of the Prostate

Unfortunately, there is another disorder of the prostate that is quite common: cancer. The diagnosis of Prostatic cancer has been on the rise in recent years. That is probably due in no small part to a better technique for diagnosing that disease by means of the P.S.A. (Prostate Specific Antigen) blood test, combined with the fact that the mean age of the male population has increased significantly due to the availability of better medical care and newer medical technologies. The annual physical examination for all men of ages fifty or older should include a rectal examination and a P.S.A. test. The P.S.A. test has led to the early discovery of many cases of prostatic cancer that would otherwise have gone undiagnosed until symptoms signaling metastasis to other parts of the body became evident.

If prostate cancer is not detected early there is a very high rate of metastasis. When cancer leaves the prostate it goes most often to bone or brain and becomes very difficult to treat. If the cancer can be treated while it is still within the prostate there is a fair chance for cure. With that in mind, there is no excuse for men over fifty not having an annual rectal examination and P.S.A. test.

Chapter Five
THE REPRODUCTIVE SYSTEM

In the previous chapter we looked at the urinary systems of males and females. Our focus was on the organs that make urine and transport urine out of the body. There was description of the organs only from the standpoint of their function in the urinary system. Now we change our focus and first look at the male organs only from the standpoint of their functions as organs of reproduction. The female organs of reproduction will then be discussed m great detail.

THE MALE REPRODUCTIVE SYSTEM

The male reproductive organs include the penis, the prostate, with its seminal vesicles, the testicles which will be referred to as the testes, and the conduction system that is involved in transportation of the sperm cells.

The Penis

In the discussion of the urinary system we saw the penis as the structure surrounding the urethra, the final tube in the route of excretion of urine from the body. It is most certainly that, but it serves another role as the organ by which sexual penetration of the female vagina is accomplished and through which the sperm is conducted from the testes into the vagina.

During the act of urination and for most of a male's waking and sleeping hours the penis is a soft, flexible structure varying from two or three inches to five inches in length. During the state that is referred to in medical terms as "tumescence", or more commonly as "an erection" the penis can be six to eight inches in length, and quite rigid, enabling deep penetration into the vagina. How does this transformation occur? It is a very complex process that we take for granted until there is a problem. That process is worth some discussion.

The penis is richly supplied with arteries and veins that have the function of bringing blood in and taking blood out, as in all parts of the body. In addition there are very large veins, distributed on both sides of the penis. There are specialized muscles within the penis that have the function of acting as valves on the arteries and veins, allowing arterial blood to enter the large veins of the penis, causing an erection. Those muscles allow blood to flow into the penis, and also restrict the outflow of blood from the veins. Those veins fill with blood, causing the erection to occur. It is an efficient hydraulic system. That process is under the control of the autonomic nervous system, also called the "unconscious" or "involuntary" system, which is not subject to voluntary control, but can be initiated by cerebral function, such as sexual fantasies that lead to arousal. After ejaculation the muscles relax, allowing the blood to flow out of the veins, permitting detumescence to occur.

Beginning in the pre-teen years when the male is sexually stimulated, often by having sexual fantasies, the autonomic nervous system comes into play and the phenomenon of erection begins. It is quite common for that to occur during sleep, resulting in nocturnal erections and even ejaculation, referred to as "wet dreams."

The Prostate and Seminal Vesicles

The prostate was discussed at some length in the previous chapter, and will not be mentioned as part of the reproductive system except to say that its firmness and bulk, located at the base of the penis, acts as a stabilizing base in the act of intercourse.

The seminal vesicles empty into the lumen of the urethra. They manufacture and store the fluid called semen, which is secreted into the urethra at the time of ejaculation. The semen acts as a vehicle to transport sperm cells (made in the testes) through the urethra and out of the penis. That fluid is called the ejaculum.

It is a rarity to encounter any dysfunction of the seminal vesicles, other than their incidental infection because of an infection of the urethra and the prostate. Such infection is called seminal vesiculitis. The treatment of that condition is much the same as the treatment for prostatitis and urethritis.

The Testicles (Testes)

These are paired structures that are suspended beneath the perineum in a sac called the scrotum. The perineum is that space between the base of the penis and the rectum and between the female's vagina and her rectum. The testes are the essential male organ. They produce two extremely important substances: sperm cells and the male hormone, testosterone. They are egg-shaped solid organs, variable in size, but somewhere in the neighborhood of one and one-half inches in length and three- fourths of an inch in diameter to twice or three times that size, depending on the size of the person and his inherited characteristics. The testes contain millions of tiny tubes, called tubules. The tubules are packed with sperm cells in various stages of maturation. The cells of the stroma, the tissue between the tubules, form glands that manufacture the hormone testosterone.

Sperm cells are specialized cells that carry the genetic material of a male. At the time of his birth every male has his full complement of sperm cells that will last to the end of his reproductive life. Nothing that happens to him throughout his life will change that genetic material except for the possibility of his being exposed to some type of high energy radiation that might cause a mutation to occur in the genetic material of his sperm. That would be extremely rare. There is a popular misconception that lifetime experiences can alter the nature of the genetic material that a man can pass on to his offspring. That is simply not true. The sperm cells remain immature and inactive from the time of birth to the age of puberty. Then, under the influence of hormones from the pituitary gland and testosterone from the stromal cells of the testes the sperm cells begin to mature. An adolescent male, in his preteen years has the capability of inseminating a female, and initiating pregnancy.

Sperm cells in great quantities leave the testes and travel through paired tubes, each called a vas deferens, to the seminal vesicles, where they are stored. At the time of ejaculation the sperm cells, in a medium of semen, are transported to the urethra. The semen, then loaded with sperm cells, travels through the penis, and if vaginal penetration has occurred, releases its load of sperm cells which can swim upstream with their long tails and possibly encounter and penetrate the female's ovum, (egg), thus initiating a pregnancy.

Testosterone is a hormone that affects virtually every part of the male's body. Under its influence the adolescent boy undergoes changes that we associate with manhood. Facial hair appears, as well as hair in the armpits and on the body in general. The voice deepens and the body musculature becomes masculine in appearance. An additional change is in the sexual organs. The penis enlarges and pubic hair appears. The sperm cells as stated above become active under the combined influence of the hormones of the pituitary gland and testosterone. Another stage in his life has begun.

DISORDERS OF THE MALE REPRODUCTIVE SYSTEM

Infertility

Infertility in a male can be due to sperm that is in some way incapable of fertilizing an ovum. An example of that would be hypogonadism, in which the testes do not produce adequate or active sperm cells, or a history of mumps orchitis, (the involvement of the testes in a prior mumps infection), causing permanent damage to the genesis of healthy sperm. There are also frequent problems of incompatibility between the man's sperm and the woman's ovum.

Another problem commonly seen is some difficulty in the transport of sperm from the testes through the vas deferens to the urethral outlet, (meatus). Probably the most common of those is the condition called varicocele; a bagging-out of the vas deferens, causing pooling of semen within the dilated portion. That kind of problem is usually remediable by surgery. These problems and others have given rise to a large body of medical specialty techniques designed to deal with male infertility. That specialty is called andrology. Artificial insemination, using healthy sperm from a sperm donor that is inserted into the vagina and cervix of a woman during her time of ovulation has been quite successful in initiating pregnancy. Another commonly used technique is to harvest ova from a woman at the time of ovulation, and to mix them with sperm from a male donor, either the spouse or another donor in a laboratory. If successful fertilization occurs the fertilized ovum is then implanted into the uterus of the female, or of a "surrogate mother" selected in advance, to be carried throughout the pregnancy. Those techniques have been in use for many years with good results.

Erectile Dysfunction

As described above penile erection is a very complicated process. It depends on the proper functioning of many parts of the body, all operating at a level below consciousness. First there is the requirement that there is a good blood supply to the penis. That can be lessened by a number of problems: a congenital abnormality or atherosclerotic changes that narrow the caliber of the arteries. Diabetes can accelerate the atherosclerotic process, affecting erectile function.

There is another factor that can interfere with the process of erection. That is malfunction of the autonomic nervous system that either prevents the attainment of an erection or interrupts the process, causing premature detumescence or premature ejaculation. In most cases the latter problem is related to unconscious psychological processes that can deny the individual the erection that he ostensibly wants to have. Of all the possible causes of erectile dysfunction that is the one most often seen. In most cases psychotherapy offers some degree of improvement in sexual function.

There is reason to be hopeful for relief of this problem due to the advent of medications; such as Viagra and its successors, that can override the autonomic dysfunction and allow a good erection to occur. Quite often after several successful episodes of intercourse with the help of one of those medications the individual finds that he can have normal erections because "nothing succeeds like a little success."

There are other forms of treatment for erectile dysfunction, depending upon the specific cause of that problem. Some surgical procedures are effective to shunt blood into restricted arteries, allowing erection to occur. Various splints and prostheses have been employed with varying degrees of success.

THE FEMALE REPRODUCTIVE SYSTEM

The Vagina

The labia, or lips, of the vagina, surround the entryway to the vagina. There are two pairs of these structures. The outermost are called the labia majora. They are soft, fleshy structures with skin covering and hair growth on their outer aspects. Their main function is to cushion and protect the entrance to the vagina. Lying just within the labia majora are the labia minora. These are thin, soft liplike structures. The labia majora close only incompletely, but the labia minora close completely to truly cover the entrance to the vagina.

The vagina is a tube that is lined with mucous membrane that has a profusion of mucus-producing glands. Lying outside of the mucus membrane are strong muscles, part of the muscle complex that extends from the tailbone, (coccyx), behind to the pubic bones in front. That muscle group is called the pubo-coccygeus muscle. It is very important in the support of the vaginal wall and of the bladder. Two glandular structures, called the Bartholin glands are located on either side of the vagina just within its origin. Their function is to provide lubricating mucus at the time of intercourse.

The vagina has a blind ending at its superior or deepest end. Through the top of the vagina projects the cervix of the uterus. The muscles surrounding the vagina have the capability of squeezing down, thus grasping the phallus during intercourse, directing the semen into the opening of the cervix during ejaculation.

Located just anteriorly to the edge of the vagina is a fleshy structure called the clitoris. It is highly variable in size, but is usually about one-fourth of an inch in diameter and about one-half inch in length. The clitoris is related to the penis in that it has venous structures similar to those of the penis and is capable of achieving tumescence during sexual arousal. The clitoris has a rich supply of sensory nerves that contribute to the mechanism of orgasm.

The Uterus and the Fallopian Tubes

The cervix is the entrance to the uterus, which is often referred to poetically as "the womb." The uterus is the organ in which pregnancy occurs, and the fetus grows until the time of birth.

The uterus is a truly amazing structure. In its non-pregnant state it is about the size and shape of a medium-size avocado. During the nine months in which a fetus grows within the uterus that organ becomes large enough to enclose a baby of sometimes ten or more pounds. During pregnancy it can fill most of the abdominal cavity, pressing on all of the other organs. After delivery the uterus gradually shrinks down to near to its non-pregnant size.

The body of uterus is within the peritoneal cavity. So are two ovaries and two adjacent structures called the Fallopian tubes. Those organs will be discussed at length later in this chapter, but for now it is enough to say that although there are two ovaries, only one produces an ovum each month. The Fallopian tubes travel within the wall of the uterus, ending in the cavity of the uterus.

The uterus is composed of three layers. The innermost layer is called the endometrium. It is a thick spongy mass of cells that is very richly supplied with blood vessels.

Just outside of the endometrium is the myometrium. That is a thick layer of muscle that surrounds the entire uterus. The myometrium is capable of stretching greatly during the growth of the fetus, then contracting with enough force to push out the baby during the process of labor.

The next layer, just outside of the myometrium, is a thick fibrous sheet that is covered on the outside with a smooth layer of serous membrane. It is called the serosa. The dome of the uterus at its uppermost end is covered with a thin, smooth membrane that is contiguous with the peritoneum.

The Ovaries

The ovaries are the female counterparts of the testes of the male. They are about one inch to one and a half inches in diameter and about an inch in thickness. They have a very rich blood supply, befitting of their importance to the entire body.

The ovaries share with the testes the dual function of carrying the genetic material which will be passed along to the woman's offspring and also being an endocrine gland that produce the hormone called estrogen, the principal female hormone. At the time of a female's birth she has within her ovaries all the genetic material that she inherited from her parents. She will carry that genetic material throughout her lifetime. It cannot be changed by any event or experience during her lifetime except for the very slight possibility of intense exposure to very high- energy radiation that could cause a mutation in her genes. That possibility is so slight as to be negligible.

The genetic material of a female lies within tiny structures called ova, ovum in the singular, eggs in the vernacular. The ova are packed within both ovaries. During childhood the ova lie dormant and immature. At the time of puberty, under the influence of hormones from the pituitary gland, the ovaries begin to change. The ova begin to grow, to ripen, and to become capable of participating in the act of fertilization. Usually only one ovum at a time, in only one ovary, undergoes that process each month.

The other tissues within each ovary, surrounding the ova, comprise the stroma. The stroma becomes an active endocrine gland, producing the hormone, estrogen. Estrogen enters the blood stream and is carried throughout the body. Under its influence a girl undergoes the bodily changes that identify her as a woman. Her breasts become glandular and enlarge. Her hips and other bodily contours assume the configuration of a woman, pubic and axillary, (armpit) hair grows and the transition into womanhood occurs.

PREGNANCY

In the mature female, in most cases, only one ovary gives rise to a mature ovum each month. That ovum exists within a structure called an ovarian follicle within the ovary. Under the influence of a pituitary hormone called Follicle Stimulating Hormone, F.S.H. for short, the follicle releases its ovum which ruptures out of the ovary with considerable force.

Occasionally, after the ovum leaves the ovarian follicle it is met within the peritoneal cavity by the thousands of sperm that traversed the Fallopian tubes and have found their way upstream to that extent. If a sperm cell succeeds in penetrating the wall of the ovum fertilization occurs. The fertilized ovum then enters the adjacent Fallopian tube and makes its way through the tunnel in the wall of the uterus to nestle in the thick, nourishing endometrium to begin embryonic growth. In some cases the ovum enters the Fallopian tube before it can be fertilized, and within that tube is penetrated by a sperm in which case the fertilized ovum travels into the endometrial cavity. In even a smaller number of instances fertilization occurs within the endometrial cavity.

In rare cases the ovum is fertilized within the peritoneal cavity, but fails to make the trip into the Fallopian tube. It attaches to some adjacent structure, but soon dies there for lack of nutrition.

There are many exceptions to the above scenarios. A very common one is the production of two or more ova from the same ovary in a single month. If that occurs, and all the ova enter the Fallopian tube simultaneously there is a strong likelihood that each ovum will be fertilized by a sperm cell, and multiple fertilized ova will enter the endometrium to begin embryonic life. The result of that is the production of fraternal twins, or triplets, or more.

That scenario has become much more common since advent of the use of fertility-enhancing drugs. We quite often hear about the birth of triplets or quadruplets in women who have taken those drugs. Those babies will not be identical because multiple sperm cells fertilized multiple ova, each having different combinations of genetic material in their composition.

Another commonplace occurrence is the formation and birth of identical twins. The explanation of that phenomenon is that following fertilization of a single ovum by a single sperm cell the embryo divides into two separate embryos, each having identical genetic material from the single sperm cell. They can only develop into identical fetuses and babies.

Another exception to the first scenario is that of tubal pregnancy in which the fertilized ovum cannot pass through the Fallopian tube to reach the endometrium due to a disparity between the size of the embryo and the caliber of the Fallopian tube. That can be, in some cases, the result of a previous infection within the tube, causing scarring and narrowing of its lumen. Because the rapidly enlarging embryo exerts pressure on the wall of the Fallopian tube it causes pain, followed by fever and ultimately the signs and symptoms of peritonitis if the Fallopian tube ruptures. . That is a very serious problem requiring immediate surgery. In the course of that surgery, depending on the extent of damage to the Fallopian tube, the embryo can be extracted, preserving the tube, or the tube must be removed.

Within the ovary, after ovulation the follicle that contained the ovum that was released undergoes a change into a glandular structure called a corpus luteum. The corpus luteum begins to function as an endocrine gland. Under the influence of a pituitary hormone called luteinizing hormone, (LH) it secretes a hormone called progesterone.

Under the influence of progesterone the endometrial lining of the uterus becomes very thick and spongy, creating an ideal environment for the growth of a fertilized ovum into an embryo. The progression of fertilized ovum into embryo involves the division of cells and under the control of the genetic material in the fertilized ovum, differentiation and shaping into the earliest forms of all the organs in the body. In nine months of maturation within the uterus the embryo develops into a fetus, then into a baby.

THE MENSTRUAL CYCLE

Menstruation is a phenomenon that occurs in most females beginning at the time of puberty, usually in the early teen years. It is the body's way of cleaning out the endometrial lining of the uterus in order to prepare for the possibility of receiving and nurturing a pregnancy following the next ovulation.

In the event that fertilization of the ovum does not occur, on the fifteenth day after ovulation the corpus luteum abruptly ceases to produce its hormone, progesterone. That immediately causes a great change to occur. Deprived of progesterone, the endometrium immediately starts to break down, with the resultant discharge of blood and cast off endometrial cells into the vagina that we recognize as menstruation. In most women the bleeding lasts from five to seven days. Then, under the influence of the ovarian hormone, estrogen, the body creates a new lining of endometrial cells, building up that nice thick layer that will prepare itself for the reception of another ovum in about fifteen days.

That is the familiar menstrual cycle that will go on until around age fifty in most women. At that time the phenomenon of the menopause begins.

CONTRACEPTION (BIRTH CONTROL)

Before going on to the menopause, which is a normal and permanent change in the life of every woman, it makes good sense to discuss the various means of preventing unwanted pregnancy. There are two categories of contraception.

1. Permanent contraception, because future pregnancies would be dangerous to the mother, or to the baby, or in the case where the woman, or the man or the couple definitely desire to have no more children. In that situation the only sure way to prevent further pregnancy is surgical. The female can elect to have her Fallopian tubes cut and tied, (tubal ligation), thus preventing the possibility of any ova being fertilized. The male can elect to have a vasectomy, an operation in which the vas deferens tubes that carry sperm from the testes into the seminal vesicles are cut and the ends tied. If the male has a vasectomy the couple must use a temporary method of contraception until the male has

had several ejaculations, in order to empty the seminal vesicles of any viable sperm cells that may remain.

2. Temporary contraception, which can be discontinued, allowing pregnancies to occur in the future. There are three ways to accomplish that goal: (A) withdrawal, in which the penis is removed from the vagina before ejaculation occurs. This is an extremely uncertain method because a male cannot always withdraw in time. (B) Barrier methods, in which the male uses a condom or the female uses a diaphragm that must be inserted into her vagina prior to intercourse and left in place for twelve to twenty four hours afterward. Because of the potential for improper technique in inserting the diaphragm it is an imperfect contraceptive technique, but is much more effective than the condom in most cases. There is a possibility that the condom could come off during intercourse, or that there could be leakage of semen around the condom. The one additional advantage of the condom is that, as a barrier, it is a fairly effective means of preventing transmission of sexually transmitted diseases. That feature makes it the choice over the diaphragm in casual intercourse, where the couple cannot be certain about the sexual health of each other. To be more careful, both the condom and the diaphragm can be used simultaneously in casual intercourse.

3. The third method of temporary contraception is the one most favored by married couples and couples who know each other very well. That is the use of hormonal substances, either in the form of contraceptive pills, or injected hormones or hormonal substances that are implanted under the skin of the woman. (Both married and single women, of course, commonly use birth

control pills as a very effective way to prevent pregnancy, but in the light of the dangers of being exposed to sexually transmitted diseases in the present climate, a condom should also be used for protection.)

The way that hormonal contraception works is like this: you may recall that following ovulation the ovarian follicle, now the corpus luteum, begins to produce a hormone called progesterone. If fertilization of the ovum occurs and pregnancy follows, the corpus luteum continues to produce progesterone throughout the duration of the pregnancy. The main effect of the progesterone is to enhance the condition of the endometrium. Another effect, however is that it stops further ovulation until after the pregnancy.

In the late nineteen fifties and early sixties researchers found that if some type of hormonal substance that resembled progesterone could be introduced into the female's body ovulation could be suspended indefinitely. With no ovum being produced there is no possibility of impregnation, even though there might be sperm cells knocking at the door quite regularly.

Out of this discovery a vast industry developed. The first contraceptives were injectable long-acting forms of synthetic progesterone. Then a successful method of orally taking the progesterone-like substance, which the medical community named "a progestational agent" was found, and the first birth control pills were produced. The response of the public was overwhelming. Since those early days many varieties of "B.C. Pills" have been formulated, but the same basic concept applies to them all. They are, in general, safe, with a track record of more than forty years of use worldwide, with minimal problems.

After stopping the pills for a short time fertility returns. The pills are formulated so that normal menstrual cycles occur every month. A relatively small percentage of women prefer to have monthly injections of a long acting form of synthetic progesterone, or implantation of a solid form of a similar hormone under their skin at intervals. There does not appear to be any advantage in using either of those methods over taking B.C. pills.

The most serious complication associated with the use of hormonal contraceptives is the danger of thrombi (blood clots) in the deep veins of the legs and pelvis with the possibility of embolization of thrombi to the lungs. This is a rare, but very serious complication. The underlying reason for this phenomenon is not fully understood. Thrombosis of leg veins occurs most often in women who smoke while using hormonal contraception. That is another powerful reason for women to STOP SMOKING.

Thrombosis in leg veins is a rare complication of taking B.C. pills, but, of course, a very serious one. It does not, in the opinion of most physicians, invalidate the use of that method of contraception, but it must be stated as a possible hazard.

THE MENOPAUSE

Just as the time clock of the body switches on the female reproductive system at the time of puberty, it switches it off at an average age of fifty in most women, initiating the menopause.

The pituitary gland, which is the master endocrine gland of the body, initiates the onset of activity of the ovaries by the production and release of Follicle

Stimulating Hormone, (F.S.H.), and the phenomenon of ovulation with Luteinizing Hormone, (L.H.). The onset of menopause is caused by the pituitary's stopping the production of those hormones. The production of estrogen, the feminizing hormone, ceases. There is some inscrutable wisdom in those processes because a pre-pubertal girl is too young to have the responsibility of having and raising a baby, and a woman in her fifties is, in most cases, probably too old to have a baby and to raise that baby into adulthood.

With the onset of menopause the woman's body begins to undergo changes. When estrogen production ceases menstruation stops. Some of the physical characteristics of womanhood that we identified earlier at the time of puberty begin to change. This is highly variable from woman to woman and population to population, but there is a progressive change in all women.

Among the changes seen are the onset of hot flashes that are due to unpredictable dilatation of blood vessels, with sweating and flushing of the skin. There are changes in the skin texture and loss of calcium from the bones. There are behavioral changes. In some societies these changes are accepted as part of the normal life cycle, but in many parts of the world they are unacceptable to most women. That fact initiated vast research, leading to our next topic of discussion.

HORMONE REPLACEMENT THERAPY (HRT)

In spite of the fact that the phenomenon of menopause is a natural event, known since the beginning of recorded history, modern women have strongly disliked the hot flashes and the change in physical appearance that are a natural part of menopause.

In the nineteen fifties and sixties it was learned that the administration of estrogen, the principal female hormone, could have a remarkable effect in reducing or deferring those menopausal changes, although the process of ovulation could not be restored because of the shutting down of the pituitary production of FSH and LH.

The first medications that were marketed for menopause were composed of estrogenic substances only. The women who took them enjoyed freedom from hot flashes and felt much better. However the ongoing stimulation of the uterine endometrium caused a hypertrophic piling up of the cells of the endometrium. With no menstrual period to flush out the cells some underwent malignant degeneration. The incidence of endometrial cancer in women taking those hormones increased dramatically.

That shocking occurrence led to a re-designing of the regimen for post-menopausal hormone replacement therapy. A course of treatment was designed to mimic the actual hormonal changes of the natural menstrual cycle by taking estrogenic medication for the first fifteen days of the month, then adding a progestational medication for ten days, then stopping both medications. The estrogen supplied the body with female hormone, then adding the progesterone prepared the endometrium for menstruation, and then the stopping of both hormones caused the onset of menstrual bleeding. Five days were allowed for the menstrual period, and then the cycle began over again.

That cycle was successful in avoiding the danger of cancer of the endometrium but many women complained that they did not wish to continue having menstruation past the age of fifty.

The researchers went back to the research laboratory. The next offering was a preparation containing an estrogenic agent and a progestational agent in a single tablet, to be taken continuously month after month. The addition of a progestational agent continuously was well tolerated and safely prevented the piling-up of endometrial cells within the uterus with no stimulus or need for menstruation to occur. That regimen was widely tested in many large studies involving thousands of women and was judged to be effective and safe. It is used worldwide today.

At the time of this writing there has arisen serious question about the safety of post-menopausal use of female hormones. The most serious objection is the possibility that the hormones are responsible for an increased incidence of breast cancer in women who are taking them. Most practicing physicians are continuing to prescribe H.R.T., although there is a mounting body of evidence that H.R.T. does increase the risk of heart attack in women. On the other side of the coin there is evidence that hormone replacement therapy confers benefits, protecting women from other illnesses, notably osteoporosis. The jury is still out, but the prescription of replacement female hormones is definitely on the wane.

DISORDERS OF THE FEMALE REPRODUCTIVE SYSTEM

DISORDERS OF THE VAGINA

The vaginal introitus (the labia and the vaginal opening) is subject to traumatic injury from bruising, scratching or scraping, usually sustained through some type of athletic or sexual activity. That is usually painful and frequently accompanied by some degree of bleeding, but rarely is a serious problem.

Vaginal infections are extremely common. Such infections are usually referred to as "vaginitis." Yeast-type fungal infections, usually due to an organism called candida are seen from infancy to old age. Yeast organisms are always present within the vagina, but do not cause an infection. The cause is often some type of change in the vaginal environment. An extremely common cause is the use of antibiotic medication for any infection in the body. Antibiotics can incidentally destroy the normal bacterial flora of the vagina. That flora usually is protective against opportunistic infection from the yeast in the environment. Severe itching, redness and swelling of the mucosal lining and a cheesy white thick discharge often signal yeast infections. Those infections can usually be treated by the application of topical medications, or by a single oral dose of a prescription medication.

Bacterial infections are also quite commonly seen. They are most often the result of sexual activity in which there is inadvertent transfer of secretions from the patient's own rectal area into her vagina. The bacterial flora of the digestive tract, present on the perianal skin is extremely infectious to the vagina. A much more serious cause of vaginitis is a sexually transmitted disease, STD. Such diseases can be of bacterial origin, such as syphilis, or gonorrhea, or of viral origin, most seriously due to the HIV virus.

There is always the risk of the male partner becoming infected with an already present organism within the vagina. For the protection of both partners it is my most sincere advice to use a condom during casual intercourse.

Another common vaginal problem involves the Bartholin glands that are located within the vaginal lining. They are lubricating glands, secreting thick mucus. The duct of one of those glands can become blocked, preventing the outflow of mucus. Bacterial infection of the gland then follows, with pain and fever. The usual treatment is some type of surgery to drain the gland, and the use of antibiotics, with generally good results.

DISORDERS OF THE UTERINE CERVIX

Ascending from the vagina we come to the cervix of the uterus. Infections of the cervix with organisms that infect the vagina are quite common. Such infections are called cervicitis. Most cases of cervicitis are technically S.T.D. because they are caused by sexual activity. In most cases cervicitis is treated with topical medications, and oral antibiotics, with good results.

The cervix is a common site for cancerous change. As in the case of most cancers there is no known cause, but there is a relationship between a vaginal infection caused by a virus called Human Papilloma Virus, or H.P.V. virus and cervical cancer. Cervical cancer is usually diagnosed by the technique called Pap. Smear, named after its originator; doctor Papanicolaou. The technique of Pap. Smear is very simple, and painless. The examiner looks inside the vagina with an instrument called a vaginal speculum, and in most cases can see the cervix. A small wooden paddle is wiped across the cervix, collecting cells from the tip of the cervix. That paddle is then wiped onto a glass slide, transferring those cells to the slide. A preservative is applied to prevent distortion of the cells, and the slide is sent to a laboratory to be examined under a microscope. By means of special staining of the cells on the slide cancer cells will "light up" and be seen very clearly microscopically. This is the most reliable and simplest of all tests for cancer.

Every adult woman should have a Pap. Smear every year to detect the earliest signs of cervical cancer, which may be quite curable by local treatment of the cervix. Untreated cervical cancer usually extends to involve the body of the uterus and can be a much more serious problem.

DISORDERS OF THE BODY OF THE UTERUS

The most commonly seen problem of the uterus involves the endometrium. Due to an imbalance of hormonal regulation of the menstrual cycle a buildup of the endometrium can occur. There is incomplete sloughing off of the thickened endometrial lining causing menstrual bleeding to continue beyond the normal five to seven days. The bleeding might last for weeks. There can be significant blood loss in some cases, resulting in anemia.

When the patient reports this to her physician there is usually an examination that determines the diagnosis of endometrial hyerplasia, which is the medical term for thickening of the endometrial tissue. The usual treatment for this condition is called dilation and curettement of the uterus. The medical shorthand is D&C. It can be performed in a short stay facility, or in the gynecologist's office. The cervix of the uterus is dilated open with an instrument and the endometrial lining is scraped out with an instrument called a curette. The procedure is moderately painful, but pain can usually be minimized with a mild anesthetic. The tissue is sent to a pathologist for microscopic examination to rule out the possibility of cancerous change of the endometrium. That treatment most often allows the endometrial cells to regain their normal thickness, and menstruation follows in a normal way.

The next most frequently seen disorder of the body of the uterus is called leiomyoma of the muscle wall of the uterus. The common name for that condition is "fibroids." This is a benign, (non-cancerous) condition in which there are multiple tumors of the muscle wall that grow inward toward the center of the uterus, as well as outward, allowing them to be felt during pelvic examination. There is usually heavy bleeding that continues after the normal duration of menstruation, causing anemia in many cases. The treatment for fibroids is frequently hysterectomy, a general term for removal of the uterus. There is another choice of treatment called myomectomy. That is a surgical procedure in which the tumors are removed from the uterus, leaving the uterus intact. That is a much more complicated surgery, and is usually reserved for women who are desirous of becoming pregnant and wish to have the uterus preserved.

Hysterectomy can be done in one of three stages:

A. Simple hysterectomy is an operation in which the uterus is removed but the cervix and the ovaries and Fallopian tubes are left intact. This is the quickest procedure, and the one that causes the least amount of trauma to the patient, and has the shortest healing time. However, since cancer of the cervix continues to be a reality even though the body of the uterus is removed, that procedure is rarely done today.

B. Complete hysterectomy involves removal of the body of the uterus and the cervix in a single unit, leaving the ovaries and the Fallopian tubes intact. That procedure is often done in the case of young women to avoid a premature menopause.

C. Total hysterectomy, in which the body of the uterus and the cervix are removed as a unit, and the ovaries and Fallopian tubes are also removed. That procedure is done as a precautionary measure in women who are close to, or beyond the age of menopause to prevent possible future ovarian cancer.

In the event of total hysterectomy removal of the ovaries causes abrupt loss of the hormone, estrogen. That loss creates a state of premature menopause which is a severe shock to the woman's body. In that case hormone replacement with estrogen is usually instituted immediately.

DISORDERS INVOLVING THE FALLOPIAN TUBES

There are two kinds of problems that commonly involve the Fallopian tubes. The most frequently seen is infection. That is always secondary to infections of the vagina that enter the uterus and find the opening of one or both Fallopian tubes, and travel upward. That kind of infection is labeled Pelvic Inflammatory Disease, or PID. It is almost always a severe infection with fever, peritonitis and severe abdominal pain. The patient is quite often hospitalized for intensive treatment with antibiotics.

In spite of that treatment the end result is often extensive scaring of the involved tube, causing complete or partial closure of that tube. If both tubes are involved the patient can lose the capability of having normal fertilization of her ovum because either due to the scarring the sperm are incapable of reaching and fertilizing the ovum or the ovum, if fertilized, is incapable of passing through to the endometrium.

With modern techniques of in vitro fertilization it is possible for a woman to have her ovum removed at the time of ovulation by laparoscopic technique. The ovum is then fertilized in the laboratory by her partner's sperm cells, and then implanted into the patient's own uterus. That procedure is called in- vitro fertilization, or IVF. That is a difficult and expensive technique, but it presents the possibility of having a baby with the woman's own ovum and the partner's own sperm cells.

The next most common disorder involving the Fallopian tube is called tubal pregnancy. That condition was described in detail in the chapter on Pregnancy.

DISORDERS OF THE OVARIES

A rare disorder is ovarian agenesis, which means some type of genetic or fetal disorder that causes the ovary, or ovaries to be absent or poorly formed. That condition is extremely complicated to manage, requiring the combined talents of several medical disciplines.

Another rare disorder is malfunction or premature shutting down of ovarian function due to a defect in the pituitary gland, resulting in deficiency of the hormones FSH and LH. The ovaries are otherwise remarkably free of problems from the time of puberty to the time of menopause, with the exception of two conditions that are, unfortunately quite common.

The first of those is hemorrhagic ovulation. That condition, called "mittelschmerz" by early German surgeons, was described in detail in the section on Acute Appendicitis earlier in this text, but it will be reviewed briefly here. Hemorrhagic ovulation occurs mainly in girls and young women. At the time of ovulation the ovum bursts forth from the capsule of the ovary with considerable force. There is bleeding into the peritoneal cavity probably from the ovarian follicle, causing acute peritonitis. If the ovulation is on the right side the symptoms can mimic those of acute appendicitis. It is not uncommon for exploratory surgery to be performed at that time to prevent missing the very critical diagnosis of acute appendicitis. Such surgery should in no way affect adversely the future functioning of the ovary, or the ability to have children.

The second, and most serious problem affecting the ovaries follows.

Ovarian Cancer

Ovarian cancer is, unfortunately, quite frequently seen. At the beginning it is a "silent" disorder, because there are no early symptoms. The first sign of its presence is quite often the finding of a distant metastasis in bone, brain, liver or other tissues. There is no easy cure for this dreadful disease. The best that medicine can offer at this point in time is a chance for very early detection by means of annual pelvic examinations. There is considerable difference of opinion among physicians about the use of a blood test called CA-125 as a screening test for ovarian cancer. The chief objection is that there is a reasonable possibility of having a false positive or false negative result of that test. In the event of a positive CA-125 test, because of the potential seriousness of a true positive result, it is necessary to do very extensive follow-up studies to search for more evidence of the cancer or its metastases. The required tests are quite expensive, and usually require some kind of surgical procedure. It is an extremely difficult decision to forego the CA-125 as a screening test. I could not offer a solution to that dilemma, although my personal professional choice was to order the study more often than not.

If the patient is found to have true ovarian cancer, determined by tissue biopsy a thorough series of tests must be done to try to identify the presence of extension of the cancer to adjacent structures or of distant metastases. If those are found the patient should have complete removal of all of her pelvic organs. Following that some plan must be made for treating the metastases. She must be followed with frequent examinations to rule out new evidence of metastases. If the patient is found to have evidence of distant metastases she should still have total abdominal hysterectomy.

Ovarian cancer is a very sad disease because so many young women are afflicted with it and the likelihood of cure is not very good. This fact strongly enforces the need for an annual pelvic examination performed by a competent physician or gynecologist, even though the earliest signs of the disease may not be evident at that particular point in time.

THE BREASTS

Although the breasts are not a part of the reproductive system they are so closely allied to the concept of femininity, and to the functioning of the reproductive system that they are properly addressed in this section.

The Male Breast

Males have breasts. In most males they do not develop under the influence of hormones into milk-forming organs, but under certain conditions their nipples secrete a clear, gray liquid called colostrum. That is probably due to response to the stimulation of a pituitary hormone called lactogenic hormone. The production of colostrum is usually a brief phenomenon, but can sometimes be of long duration. The condition usually subsides spontaneously.

Male nipples have the same supply of sensory nerves as do females'. They are sensitive to stimulation and have the capability of becoming erect.

Male breasts share with female breasts the propensity for developing malignant tumors, although the incidence is much lower in males. The treatment of that very rare condition is essentially the same as that in the case of women.

The Female Breast

Anatomically the female breast is quite similar to that of the male. Both are situated anteriorly to the pectoralis major muscle on each side of the chest. There is a nipple situated in approximately the middle of each. Within the breast the nipple is joined to a system of milk ducts which are connected to milk glands. With the proper hormonal stimulation those glands manufacture milk and secrete that milk into ducts that carry the milk to the nipple. The difference between the male and the female breast lies in the fact that the female breast changes at the time of puberty into a structure that can do all of those things, but the male breast, lacking the stimulation of female hormones does not.

The female breasts are quite small until the onset of puberty. Then, under the influence of estrogen hormone from the ovary they enlarge. Their enlargement is partly due to enlargement of the milk glands and partly to infiltration of the tissues with fat. Enlargement of the breasts can continue for most of a lifetime if the woman has the tendency to accumulate fat in her breasts, although many women have small breasts throughout their lifetime.

The greatest stimulus to the enlargement of the breasts is pregnancy. At the time of delivery the pituitary gland is stimulated to manufacture and secrete a hormonal substance called lactogenic hormone, (L.H.). Carried through the blood stream from the pituitary to the breasts that hormone stimulates the breast glands to enlarge and to start manufacturing milk. After the birth, if the baby is permitted to nurse that stimulation keeps the breasts producing milk until nursing is discontinued. When nursing stops the flow of milk stops, and the milk glands gradually shrink. The breasts may remain enlarged, or return to their pre-pregnancy size, or even becomes smaller than in the pre-pregnant state.

DISORDERS OF THE FEMALE BREAST

There is a very common tendency in many women for the breasts to become fibrous and to develop cystic changes in the milk ducts. That is due to the monthly changes within the breasts in response to the cyclical production of female hormones by the pituitary gland.

There is associated inflammation that results in fibrous and cystic changes. This causes breast soreness, tenderness, and the formation of "lumpy breasts." There is no evidence that this condition predisposes to serious breast disease. There are two disorders of a more serious nature that are very commonly seen in women: mastitis and breast cancer.

Mastitis is the name given to infection within the breast. It is usually due to an irritation and inflammation of the nipple with bacterial infection that then extends inwardly to involve the duct system and the inner tissues of the breast. The breast becomes painful, red and swollen. Pus may issue from the nipple. The patient develops fever and chills, and is very sick. . In most cases mastitis can be effectively treated with antibiotics. Surgery is sometimes required to drain cystic abscesses.

Breast Cancer

The incidence of reported breast cancer has increased dramatically in the last half of the twentieth century, and into the twenty first century. That fact is due in large part to the earlier detection of that disease by means of routine screening mammography. Very early cancers of the breast can be seen on mammogram X-Ray, long before they can be felt. As a result of that technique many women have had curative surgery performed. In pre-mammogram days the cancer could not be diagnosed until it was large enough to be felt. That period of time often allowed for extensive invasion of the breast and the adjacent lymph nodes, and metastasis to remote areas of the body. The recent innovation of digital mammography has increased the ability to make early diagnosis of breast cancer.

Most breast cancers have the tendency to spread to the adjacent lymph nodes in the axilla, (armpit) and from there via the blood stream and lymph system to distant tissues in the body. Once that has occurred the chance for cure becomes very small. If a mammogram shows very early cancer, confined to the breast there is a very good chance that excision of the cancer and an area surrounding the cancer, followed by radiation to the breast itself will cure the disease. In early cases it is common to remove and examine the closest lymph nodes in the axilla adjacent to the affected breast. If the lymph nodes show no sign of invasion by the cancer there is no reason for additional treatment. In past years, for more advanced cases, removal of the breast, (mastectomy), followed by removal of the axillary lymph nodes and post-operative radiation had been standard practice. Modern treatment usually avoids removal of the breast in favor of radiation and chemotherapy which often achieve the same goal while preserving the breast.

As in the case of most cancers, there is no definite known cause for breast cancer. Self-examination is an excellent habit, but this writer believes firmly that annual breast examination and mammograms for all women over thirty should be done. There is no danger from the X-radiation, which is a very small dose, and the benefits of early diagnosis and treatment are enormous.

Chapter Six
THE ENDOCRINE SYSTEM

OVERVIEW

There are in general two kinds of glandular organs, exocrine and endocrine. Exocrine organs consist of structures of glands that produce chemical substances that are secreted to perform functions that occur in close proximity to those glands. Examples of exocrine glands are the sweat glands and oil glands in the skin and the glands within the stomach that secrete acid and digestive enzymes. Endocrine glands are organs that manufacture and secrete substances called hormones. Hormones are chemical compounds that are secreted into the blood stream and are carried by the blood throughout the body. They play a major role in the development and functioning of virtually every part of the body. The endocrine glands are:

The pituitary
The thyroid
The parathyroids
The adrenals
The ovaries
The testes
The pancreas

All endocrine glands function in essentially the same way. They are composed of dense glandular cells and have very rich blood supplies. Each manufactures its own specific hormonal product or products and secretes those hormones into the blood stream in response to a signal of need from the target organs. The pancreas is actually partly an endocrine gland, and partly an exocrine gland. The endocrine portion manufactures the hormone insulin which is secreted into the blood stream and the exocrine portion manufactures the pancreatic digestive enzymes that are secreted into the duodenum to facilitate digestion of fats and sugars. The hormone cholecystokinin, manufactured within the stomach is an exception. It is secreted into the blood stream to cause the gall bladder to contract and push bile into the digestive tube to help with the digestion of fatty substances. Cholecystokinin is an endocrine hormone with a very local and specific target organ and is usually not listed as a classical endocrine hormonal.

The endocrine glands are amazingly complicated and diverse in their functioning and the stimuli that drive each of them.

We will begin with the pituitary, which is the master endocrine gland of the body.

THE PITUITARY

This gland, also called the hypophysis, controls the functions of the thyroid, adrenals, ovaries and the testes. In addition, it produces hormones that control our growth, the onset of puberty, the menstrual cycle, and the onset of lactation at the terminus of pregnancy. That is only a part of the amazing functions of the pituitary.

The pituitary is about the size of a large pea. It is divided into two portions called the anterior and posterior hypophysis. It is located within the base of the skull in a bony niche called the Sella Turcica. That name, which means "Turkish saddle", was conferred by ancient anatomists because of its resemblance to that particular horse saddle. The pituitary has a rich blood supply and extensive connections with the nervous system. In fact, the posterior portion (called the neurohypophysis) is connected by a stalk of nerve tissue to a region of the brain called the hypothalamus. The pituitary receives nerve stimulation from the brain, as well as chemical messages via the blood stream, sent from other endocrine glands. The influence of neural messages from the hypothalamus to the posterior pituitary can be seen in the over-active response of the thyroid gland to severe prolonged emotional stress states, described later in this chapter.

The anterior portion of the pituitary, called the adenohypophysis, contains a highly sensitive chemical laboratory that constantly monitors the incoming flow of blood, measuring the level of hormones from all the other endocrine glands. That information is then used to tell the anterior pituitary to manufacture and secrete hormones that stimulate each of the other endocrine organs in exactly the amount needed to ensure their proper functioning. All of this is done instantly and continuously, day and night.

As described in the previous chapter, the pituitary secretes hormones, called Follicle Stimulating Hormone, Luteinizing Hormone, and Lactogenic hormone. All of those are instrumental in the maturation and development of the sexual organs, pregnancy, the menstrual cycle, the nursing of infants, and the menopause.

The pituitary monitors the blood level of hormone from the thyroid gland. If the level is too low the pituitary secretes thyroid stimulating hormone (TSH) which travels through the blood stream to the thyroid and stimulates it to secrete more thyroid hormone. If the level of thyroid hormone is too high the pituitary stops secreting TSH until the level of thyroid hormone falls to normal. There is an exception to that process that will be discussed in depth in the section on the thyroid gland.

DISORDERS OF THE PITUITARY GLAND

There are some serious disorders that can befall the pituitary. The one that is most often seen is the development of a benign tumor, called a pituitary adenoma. That growth enlarges in size, causing the pituitary to be seriously compressed within the hard bony structure of the sella turcica. The pituitary gradually loses its ability to manufacture and secrete its vital hormones.

The first diagnostic signs are the failure of function of the target organs. Pituitary adenomas can also be responsible for over-production of pituitary hormones. Overproduction of growth hormone can produce gigantism in growing children or, in adults, a condition called acromegaly in which there is selective enlargement of the skull and jaw as well as general musculoskeletal growth. Insufficient production of growth hormone in young children can cause permanent very small stature.

Visualization of the pituitary by C.T. or MRI scans can verify the presence of the tumor. The standard therapy at this point in time is surgery to remove the tumor. That is very delicate and hazardous surgery. It is hoped that alternative treatment will be developed in the future.

Another type of disorder of the pituitary is a vascular event, such as a thrombus or ruptured arterial aneurysm that can seriously interfere with the pituitary blood supply and cause the gland to lose function. That is a calamitous event. The only therapy for that is to attempt to replace all the pituitary hormones, or the hormones of its target endocrine organs. No human or machine thus far invented can perform that job as well as this tiny pea-sized gland, but therapeutic regimens are available to attempt to replace the vital hormones.

THE THYROID

The thyroid is located in the middle of the front of the neck. There are two lobes, one on each side of the midline, connected by a narrow strand of tissue called the isthmus of the thyroid. Each of the lobes is about one to one and a half inches in diameter and about one half inch thick. It has a very rich blood supply through which it receives an input of hormones from the pituitary and discharges its own hormone to be carried throughout the body.

Thyroid hormone affects practically every part of the body by regulating its metabolism. The thyroid is sometimes referred to as "the idle adjustment of the body", alluding to that part of an automobile engine. Thyroid hormone is produced in response to stimulation from the pituitary hormone; thyroid stimulating hormone (TSH). The pituitary chemo-receptor analyzes the level of circulating thyroid hormone. If the level is too low it secretes TSH. The thyroid responds by making and secreting thyroid hormone into the circulating blood.

Virtually all of the element iodine in the entire body is contained in the thyroid gland and the circulating thyroid hormone. The thyroid produces its hormone as an organic molecule containing three atoms of iodine. That is called tri-iodo thyronine, or T-3. It is inactive in that form. Through the body's metabolism that molecule acquires another atom of iodine and becomes thyroxine, T-4, the active thyroid hormone.

DISORDERS OF THE THYROID

Hypothyroidism

Hypothyroidism means under-activity of the thyroid gland, demonstrated by a less than normal production of active thyroid hormone. It can occur in several ways. Some people are born hypothyroid as a result of an improper in-utero environment for their fetal development, usually due to the mother being hypothyroid, or to a genetic flaw. A hypothyroid baby can usually be recognized at birth or in very early infancy and replacement with thyroid hormone can be instituted.

If hypothyroidism is not recognized at birth or in infancy the individual may not survive, in rare cases, or will never have normal development. Hypothyroid children and those who survive to adulthood are small in stature, have poor muscle development, characteristically thick, wrinkled skin, and poor intellectual development. Their speech is usually slow and often slurred. That condition is called cretinism in childhood. There is a fair chance that very early treatment with thyroid hormone will enable the infant to develop normally. Severe hypothyroidism in adult life is called "myxedema."

Hypothyroidism can be acquired during one's life by an event that damages the thyroid. An Inflammatory disease of the thyroid called Hashimoto's thyroiditis is one such condition. It is classed as an auto-immune disease. There is no known specific cause. Hashimoto's thyroiditis is extremely destructive, often completely destroying the functioning of the thyroid gland. Vascular disease that reduces the blood supply to the thyroid can damage its function seriously, but is extremely rare. Any disorder that affects the pituitary gland can affect the supply of TSH, indirectly interfering with the function of the thyroid.

In most cases hypothyroidism can be treated with thyroid hormone taken orally. In the case of myxedema, which causes permanent damage throughout the body there is no chance of restoring the damage already done, but in most cases of hypothyroidism the patient can be given considerable help with thyroid hormone replacement.

Most frequently in cases of hypothyroidism, because the hormone produced by that gland is either of poor quality or insufficient quantity the thyroid gland enlarges to compensate. The individual cells enlarge, but there is no increase in the number of functioning thyroid cells. The enlarged gland is prominent in the front of the neck. Any generalized enlargement of the thyroid is called goitre. There can be goitre formation as the result of congenital hypothyroidism, or of inflammatory disorders, such as Hashimoto's thyroiditis, or juvenile thyroiditis, which is called lymphoid thyroiditis, or in cases of severe deficiency of TSH. A cause of hypothyroid goitre which was common in the past; but is now rare, is severe deficiency of iodine in the diet. That has been virtually eliminated by the availability of iodized salt which provides enough iodine to satisfy the thyroid's need for iodine.

All of the above instances of goitre are caused by states that result in deficiency of thyroid hormone and therefore thyroid under-activity. Next we will look at goitre due to thyroid over-activity.

Hyperthyroidism

Hyperthyroidism is the name given to a state of over-activity (hyperactivity) of the thyroid. It is a very common condition having few causes. A common cause is excessive production of the pituitary hormone TSH due to high neural input. The exact mechanism is not known, but hyperthyroidism is quite often associated with a prolonged period of severe emotional stress.

The most likely scenario for this phenomenon begins with the close association of the pituitary gland with the brain through its stalk of nerve fibers connecting the pituitary with the hypothalamic region. Sustained emotional stress produces a persistent state of alarm. The brain reacts by ordering the pituitary to deal with the stress. The pituitary responds by producing an excess of TSH. The thyroid responds by producing new T-3 hormone which is converted to the active hormone T-4. The thyroid gland enlarges, forming a goitre, but that goitre produces too much thyroid hormone, in contrast with the goitre of Hashimoto's disease. That is referred to as a toxic goitre because of the excess of thyroid hormone which is very damaging to the body.

The effect of too much secretion of thyroid hormone is to over-stimulate the body. The heart rate accelerates, the nervous system reacts with tremors of the hands and entire body. The patient loses weight, speech becoming more rapid.

The great danger of toxic hyperthyroidism is that it tends to become a fixed state, autonomous, and independent of pituitary control. The body behaves as an automobile with a stuck accelerator. With the greater load imposed on the cardio-vascular system heart failure or a coronary heart attack can follow. In most cases this state, called thyrotoxicosis, and also Grave's disease (after the physician who first described the condition) persists after the initial psychological emergency state subsides. There are alternative explanations of the cause of thyrotoxicosis. The final explanation has yet to be written.

Treatment of Hyperthyroidism

The ability to diagnose and treat hyperthyroidism was greatly enhanced by the discovery that iodine made radioactive, (I-131), could be mixed in the laboratory with blood serum. The radioactive iodine was found to attach to the T-3 molecule in the laboratory, just as iodine attaches to T-3 in the blood stream, forming the active thyroid hormone T-4, (called thyroxine). That discovery then enabled a means to make a "tagged" radioactive molecule of thyroid hormone that could be measured with great accuracy with a Geiger counter-type of apparatus. The amount of uptake of radioactive iodine by the thyroid molecule gives a very exact account of the amount of circulating thyroid hormone and thereby the activity of the thyroid gland. The test involves giving the patient tiny amounts of radioactive iodine, (I-131) causing no harmful effect on the body. The iodine is then taken up by the thyroid gland in the form of T-4 thyroxine. The radioactivity of the thyroid gland is then measured. That test is called the I-131 uptake test. It is the current standard of measurement of the level of thyroid activity.

Using the same technology, it was learned that giving much larger doses of radioactive iodine would deliver a very substantial amount of radiation to the thyroid. Because virtually all of the iodine in the body is concentrated within the thyroid gland, that radioactivity, concentrated in a small area, can destroy much of the hyperactive thyroid gland without affecting the rest of the body. That is now the most popular method of treatment of severe hyperthyroidism.

There is one problem with the treatment of hyperthyroidism with I-131 for which there is no apparent solution. That is the possibility of over-dosage. If too much radiation is delivered to the thyroid it can destroy its ability to make enough hormone to satisfy the needs of the body. That results in a permanent state of hypothyroidism. The remedy is for the patient to have to take a thyroid pill every day for the rest of his or her life. That, in fact, occurs quite commonly because it is very difficult to calculate the exact dose needed to effect a cure. That is really a small price to pay for the cure of that deadly disease.

There are two other methods of treating hyperthyroidism. One is the daily oral dosage of a medication that interferes with the uptake of iodine by the thyroid. That gradually reduces the ability of the thyroid to manufacture hormone. It often does not cure the disease and in most cases must be taken for a prolonged period of time. After some months most patients prefer the radioactive iodine treatment because they cannot tolerate the medications and prefer to have a permanent cure of their disorder.

The third method of treating the hyperthyroid state is by surgical removal of the thyroid. That procedure is rarely done, except in the case of a patient who cannot tolerate the radioactive iodine treatment, such as a pregnant woman whose fetus would be jeopardized by the radiation.

Thyroid Nodules

Other than the states of hypothyroidism and hyperthyroidism, the most common disorder of the thyroid is the appearance of a nodule, (mass, or lump) in the thyroid. Such nodules can be either benign or malignant. Thyroid cancer almost always appears as a small lump or nodule on the thyroid. Because the gland is so prominent in its location nodules can often be seen and felt very early in their existence. Thyroid nodules can be associated with the hyperthyroid state. When a nodule is detected it is imperative that a diagnosis must be made as soon as possible. The first test that is usually done is the radioactive iodine uptake test. If the nodule is due to thyroid hyperactivity it will take up the I-131, and will "light up" the Geiger counter apparatus. Such a nodule is termed a "hot" nodule of normal thyroid tissue. No further action is usually taken, other than to follow the nodule with occasional examinations. If the nodule does not take up the I-131 it is termed a "cold" nodule, and will be considered to be malignant until proven otherwise. The nodule will usually then be biopsied, using a "fine needle" technique, performed in the doctor's office. The tissue will be sent for microscopic examination to determine the diagnosis of cancer. If the microscopic examination proves the diagnosis of cancer a series of tests will be performed to seek out the possible presence of metastases of the cancer elsewhere in the body. Those tests usually include PET scan, Bone scan, and MRI scan. If those are negative the patient is a candidate for surgery. The currently favored procedure is total removal of the thyroid gland, followed by radiation therapy. There is a fair chance for cure with that treatment plan.

If metastases of thyroid cancer are detected a course of I-131 radiation is usually given. That is done in the hope that the radiation will destroy the remaining thyroid cancer in metastatic sites. With the thyroid totally removed the patient will be placed on thyroid hormone tablets for the rest of his or her life. The patient must be followed very closely for signs of remote recurrences.

THE PARATHYROID GLANDS

The Parathyroid glands are multiple small bodies of glandular tissue that are located adjacent to the thyroid gland or within the substance of the thyroid. They are usually four in number. The parathyroids are very important in the regulation of calcium and phosphorus metabolism, not only in the bones, but also in all tissues. The parathyroids monitor the blood for levels of calcium and phosphorus with their own chemical receptors. If those levels are found to be too low the parathyroids secrete their hormone, parathormone. That hormone causes the increased uptake of calcium from the digestive tract and the release of calcium and phosphorus from the stores in bones to restore the blood levels to normal.

DISORDERS OF THE PARATHYROID GLANDS

The most commonly encountered disorder is the accidental removal of parathyroid glandular tissue in the course of thyroid surgery. Although there are multiple small islands of parathyroid tissue, if the surgeon inadvertently removes all of the parathyroids the patient must be given parathormone and supplemental calcium for the duration of his/her lifetime.

The other serious disorder of the parathyroids is hyperparathyroidism. The presence of too much parathyroid hormone can be caused by a benign tumor called a parathyroid adenoma, or by primary overactivity of multiple parathyroid glands. The effect of those conditions is to cause excessive production or parathormone. That causes excessive mobilization of calcium and phosphorus from the intestine and the bones. When that happens two serious problems occur. The bones can become depleted of calcium, causing weakness of the entire skeleton. More immediately, however, high blood levels of calcium can cause serious disorders of all tissues of the body, especially the heart muscle, and altered neuromuscular tone.

Parathyroid adenoma and primary hyperparathyroidism are treated with surgical removal of the adenoma, or of separate parathyroid glands. In the hands of an experienced surgeon the outcome is usually satisfactory. If, in the course of that surgery too many parathyroid glands are removed the patient must be maintained on lifetime parathormone and calcium replacement.

THE ADRENAL GLANDS

These are paired organs, each lying atop a kidney in the retroperitoneal space. The adrenals look somewhat like a fool's cap, usually about one to two inches at the base, coming to a point. As in the case of other endocrine organs they are composed of glandular cells that are richly supplied with blood vessels. The adrenals have two sections, similar to the kidneys: the outer section is called the cortex, and the inner section, the medulla.

It is quite likely that of all the endocrine glands the adrenals are the best known to most readers because of their hormonal products. The adrenal cortex is the source of corticosteroid hormones, one of which is the famous cortisone, technically called cortisol. The adrenal medulla produces another famous hormone, adrenaline, properly named epinephrine, (because it comes from an organ located on top of the kidney, remember, "Nephron"?).

The adrenal cortex has a very rich blood supply that receives continuous messages from the pituitary. The pituitary hormone that stimulates the adrenal cortex is called Adrenocorticotrophic Hormone, which is abbreviated to ACTH. The pituitary's monitoring laboratory appraises the level of the two types of adrenal cortical hormones, called glucocorticoids and mineral corticoids, and if there is need for more, sends ACTH to the adrenals to stimulate the secretion of more corticosteroids.

The adrenal medulla is richly supplied with nerve fibers from the autonomic nervous system. That system receives some of its messages from the brain, and some from the peripheral nervous system. In the case of need for stimulation of the body, for example because of a severe stress situation, the autonomic nerves stimulate the adrenal medulla to secrete epinephrine. That hormone causes the heart rate to increase, the blood pressure to rise, and the rate of metabolism of most bodily tissues to increase. It is part of the defense system of the body, preparing the body for "flight, or fight."

DISORDERS OF THE ADRENAL CORTEX

Overproduction of Corticosteroids

There are two reasons why the adrenal cortex would over-produce its hormones: either a tumor of the pituitary gland, causing an overproduction of ACTH that causes the overproduction of corticosteroids, or a tumor of the adrenal cortex itself, causing it to over-produce its hormones. The result of that oversupply of corticosteroids is a severe disorder named Cushing's disease, after the very famous physician, Harvey Cushing, who first described the condition. The oversupply of those hormones causes severe elevation of the blood pressure, the increase of weight due to both excess fat, and retained salt and water. This leads to a change of appearance, most conspicuous in the face, neck, and upper body, and to progressive increase of blood pressure. If untreated, Cushing's disease leads to death. The treatment is to find the tumor that causes the problem and to remove it. That can be very difficult, often requiring very sensitive surgery on the pituitary gland, deep in the sella turcica of the skull. It is, however, a treatable disease, and curable in many cases.

Adrenocortical Insufficiency

Failure of the adrenal cortex to manufacture an adequate supply of its corticosteroids is due to some disease process that damages the adrenal cortex, or some failure of the pituitary gland's ability to secrete ACTH. That condition is much less often seen than is Cushing's disease. The result is an individual who is thin, deficient in muscle tissue and in fat and quite often deeply tanned, due to changes in the skin pigment. It has a name: Addison's disease. This condition can be treated provided a diagnosis is made and treatment of the cause is done. Replacement of the missing hormones on a daily basis is required. The treatment of Addison's disease requires exceptional attention from skillful physicians, most often by endocrinologists.

DISEASES OF THE ADRENAL MEDULLA

The Hyperadrenal Stress State

The adrenal medulla is richly supplied with nerves from the autonomic nervous system. Acting upon signals from the higher part of the brain (cerebrum) those nerves stimulate the adrenal medulla, telling it that a stressful condition exists, and stimulating it to produce and secrete adrenaline, (epinephrine), during times of emergency or stress. Adrenaline causes the heart rate and blood pressure to rise. It causes shunting of blood away from the skin and digestive tract, and into the muscles, the heart, and the brain to prepare the body to deal with the emergency by either running away or fighting. That has been aptly dubbed the "fight, or flight

Reaction", or the alarm reaction. That might have been very important in helping our ancestors to deal with saber tooth tigers and it certainly helps us in dealing with emergencies requiring quick physical responses. It is quite likely that all of us have been frightened or angered, and have experienced our hearts pounding, the pulse racing and the skin turning pale and cool. The reason for the skin becoming cold and pale is that the alarm reaction triggered by the autonomic nervous system caused blood to be diverted from the enormous vascular bed of the skin into the muscles and the cardiovascular system to enable one to flee or fight.

That is a wonderful defense mechanism for temporarily dealing with emergencies, but it has a very serious down-side. Many people experience that sort of alarm reaction very regularly, perhaps many times each day. That can be due to living very stressful lives in their daily environment, or having a chronic anxiety state within their personal psyche that keeps the alarm reaction running continuously. The result of living in that state over a prolonged period of time is severe wear and tear stress on numerous parts of the body. The stomach, and other parts of the digestive system are deprived of their normal blood supply, the peristaltic activity is increased, causing frequent loose stools, or severe constipation alternating with diarrhea, sustained high blood pressure, and physical and nervous exhaustion. The management of that state requites skilled medical care, and possibly psychiatric care. The consequences of untreated adrenal hyperactivity can be very severe.

Over-activity of the adrenal medulla due to specific disease states is a rarity. Tumors of the adrenal medulla can cause under-production of epinephrine, but that is also a rarity.

THE OVARIES AND THE TESTES

These organs were discussed in considerable depth in the sections on the female and male organs of reproduction. Their functions as endocrine organs were also covered thoroughly, including the menstrual cycle, contraception, and the menopause. The reader is referred to that chapter for that information, rather than to have it repeated here.

THE PANCREAS AND DIABETES MELLITUS

In an earlier chapter on the digestive system the pancreas was discussed chiefly as the source of digestive enzymes. That function is extremely important but the pancreas has another vital function as well. It is the source of insulin, the hormone that regulates the metabolism of sugar in every organ of the body.

Within the body of the pancreas there are highly specialized cells called beta cells. They form clumps of tissue that are called the islets of Langerhans. Those cells produce insulin which is taken up by the many veins within the pancreas and distributed throughout the body. The pancreas is not dependent upon hormonal signals from the pituitary, but has its own sensing mechanism that measures the level of sugar in the blood. If the blood sugar becomes too high the normal pancreas produces and secretes insulin. That hormone causes the body's tissues to metabolize the sugar more rapidly, returning the blood level to a normal range. If the blood sugar level falls too low the pancreas releases less insulin, allowing the blood sugar to rise to a normal range.

Diabetes Mellitus

This disease, in which the body's ability to metabolize sugar is impaired, is technically called Diabetes Mellitus. There are basically two mechanisms that can cause diabetes to occur. The first is that the pancreas does not produce enough insulin, or that the insulin produced is abnormal and ineffective. The second mechanism that can cause diabetes is that the body's tissues can become resistant to the effect of insulin. The latter is currently the leading cause of the worldwide epidemic of diabetes. That is closely related to the epidemic increase of severe obesity which causes insulin resistance. Diabetes has become a major epidemic disease, and with it there is a shocking increase in the number of new cases of juvenile diabetes in children.

Because of either of those two mechanisms the body loses its ability to metabolize sugar. If that condition goes uncorrected the body, in effect, starves in the midst of plenty, as sugar is the chief nutrient to provide energy. When the body becomes unable to use sugar it turns to protein and fat for its sources of energy. The breakdown products of that metabolic change are toxic to the body. The body excretes un-metabolized sugar and other abnormal metabolites in order to reduce the load of toxic products. That requires an increase in the volume of urine needed to excrete the increased waste products through the kidneys. Because of that an increased need for water intake is created. Increased thirst and increased frequency and volume of urination, combined with an increased appetite, but usually loss of weight follows. Those are the hallmarks of diabetes. To repeat: Increased urination, increased thirst and drinking fluids, increased appetite and volume of eating, but paradoxical weight loss because of inability to metabolize the carbohydrates taken in.

The main effects of those metabolic changes are seen in the atherosclerotic changes in the small blood vessels of the body, chiefly in the lower extremities, the heart, the kidneys, and the eyes. As the disease continues the larger blood vessels become obstructed with atherosclerosis.

Diabetes is currently classified into two categories: insulin dependent, called Type One Diabetes and non-insulin dependent, called Type Two Diabetes. The earlier designations, juvenile onset and adult onset diabetes are now obsolete, and are no longer applicable to the current view of the disease.

In the year 2002 diabetes was declared by the World Health Organization to be an epidemic disease, chiefly of children, but also of adults. The reason is OBESITY. In the United States and in many countries throughout the world people are eating more and exercising less. Certainly, a good part of the reason for that is the profusion of electronic devices in the home. More children watch television or play electronic games as a substitute for exercise, and eat while doing it. That certainly applies to adults as well as to children. Computers are immensely attractive. Both children and adults spend hours daily at their keyboards instead of playing outdoor games or exercising in general. Fast foods, high in fats and carbohydrates and low in protein, minerals and vitamins have replaced traditional "healthy meals" in many homes. There is no other reason available to explain the epidemic status of diabetes today. It is a very serious medical and sociologic problem.

To describe the treatment of diabetes in a nutshell, people with insulin-dependent diabetes require insulin, which is given by injection to control their sugar metabolism. They are classed as "type one, or insulin-dependent diabetics." Insulin is available in many forms, most of which are self-injected by the patient at prescribed intervals. Insulin pump apparatus is used for people with very sensitive needs for insulin. That apparatus measures the individual's blood sugar levels and meters out small doses of insulin continuously.

There has been great advancement in the use of whole pancreas from cadaver donors to be implanted within the abdomen of an insulin-dependent diabetic. It is quite successful in assisting in the management of sensitive diabetics. The problem of tissue rejection of the donated pancreas is one of the chief drawbacks.

People who can be controlled with a regimen of diet and exercise plus oral medications are classed as "type two or non-insulin-dependent diabetics." In actuality, the children who are becoming diabetic because of obesity are in the same classification as those with the old adult onset diabetes, type two. It is quite common for those people classed as type two diabetics to require insulin injections from time to time to help regulate their disease. People with both types of diabetes also require strict diet control and plenty of exercise.

The cornerstone of all medical management of diabetes is to educate the patients to lose weight, to exercise regularly and to maintain that behavior for the rest of their lives. Healthy food choices are essential.

Diabetes is a very serious, and in many cases preventable disease. If those people in the world who are frankly obese could eat less and exercise more the number of people with diabetes would be markedly reduced. It is really a matter of making the personal effort. However, the effort to stop the epidemic must begin at home. It is the parents' responsibility to get their children away from their TV sets, electronic games and computers and to encourage them to participate in some type of sport or regular exercise. Children must eat properly and that diet begins at home. The huge number of fat adults must somehow be made to realize that they are eating themselves into an early grave.

NEW DIRECTIONS IN THE TREATMENT OF DIABETES

As a means of dealing with the major pandemic of obesity in the "developed nations of the world", and as a new tool in the treatment of diabetes, a recent (2006) new therapeutic approach has evolved. Drugs that work at the level of the brain to reduce the desire to eat by creating an early sense of satiety have been tested with some success in achieving weight loss in diabetics. It is too soon to make a general statement, but it would appear that there is a place for such a drug to be used by individuals who "just can't help eating a lot." The drugs are still in research trials and quite likely would be very expensive, but it is encouraging to see that such efforts are being made to treat this severe disease.

Another therapeutic tool to enable weight loss is the practice of surgically reducing the capacity of the stomach by means of permanent surgery and also by removable devices. Also, of altering the direction of the passage of digesting food to bypass the path of maximal absorption is being used. Such surgery is reserved for individuals who are grossly overweight, in the region of 100 pounds or more.

HYPOGLYCEMIA

That is the name given to the condition of low blood sugar. It can occur as a rare occasional event, due to going too long without nutrition. Most readers have probably experienced the symptoms. They include hunger, shakiness, sweating and weakness, perhaps with difficulty in concentrating and thinking. In most cases the symptoms can be reversed by eating, or taking in sugar in some form.

Hypoglycemia occurs in diabetics who take their insulin or oral medication then do not eat as their blood sugar level drops. In that case the consequences can be very severe with loss of consciousness and even coma. The patient must take in some form of readily available sugar as soon as possible. It is much safer to have a temporary rise in blood sugar than even a brief episode of hypoglycemia. The treatment for insulin-induced coma is to give intravenous sugar and mineral replacement as soon as possible.

Another cause for severe hypoglycemia is the presence of an insulin-secreting tumor of the pancreas. That is a very rarely seen tumor. The treatment is surgical removal of the tumor.

Chapter Seven
THE NERVOUS SYSTEM

OVERVIEW

The nervous system has three divisions: the central nervous system, consisting of the brain and the spinal cord, the peripheral nervous system, consisting of all of the sensory and motor nerves that lie outside of the brain and spinal cord, and the autonomic nervous system that includes elements of both the central and the peripheral nervous systems.

A good way to envision the nervous system is to think of it as a giant super-computer that can probably our-perform any computer yet designed. At the heart of the computer is the brain which continuously receives information from the outside world and the entire body via the peripheral nerves. That information comes from the outside world via the special senses that will be discussed in the next chapter and from the body itself by way of the internal sensors that monitor every part of the body continuously, day and night.

The third component of the nervous system that incorporates elements of both the central and the peripheral nervous systems is called the autonomic nervous system. Synonyms for that system are the involuntary, or the unconscious nervous system, or the vegetative nervous system. The autonomic system has profound effects on our bodies that seem to occur spontaneously, but actually represent the integration of our unconscious minds and our physical beings. It can also be thought of as a monitor or internal gyroscope that functions to keep us on course without our conscious awareness or our volitional control.

With that introduction we will begin our anatomic and physiologic tour of the nervous system, starting with the brain.

THE BRAIN

The brain has the capacity to receive multiple incoming pieces of information simultaneously. That information is then relayed by the vast internal nerve network of the brain to its memory center. The brain has virtually unlimited memory capacity. The more educated it is, the more bits of information it can store. It is quite likely that any information ever sent to the memory center is permanently stored there for the lifetime of the individual. The ability to access and process that information is highly variable from person to person, and is an important part of what is referred to as our intelligence level.

From the memory bank the bits of information are then relayed to the association center. In the association center the incoming information is compared with the stored information from the memory bank. Based on the ability to associate that incoming information with the stored information, recognition occurs and the process of judgment can go forward. The level of functioning of the association center is equally important as that of the memory center in determining the intelligence of an individual.

Judgment within the association center of the brain results in the decision to do something with the incoming information and what to do with it, or merely to keep it in the memory bank, possibly for future use.

Based on the decision reached by the association center, messages are sent to a specific part of the nervous system to take action. That action may be in the form of a muscular movement, or speech, or any action of which the body is capable.

All of these very complicated processes take place in milliseconds of time, and may involve a number of simultaneous decisions and actions. A very simple illustration would be that of a person touching a very hot object. The part of the special senses that perceives touch and heat sends the incoming message to the brain. The message is forwarded to the memory center which recognizes heat and those messages are sent on to the association center which processes that information and makes the judgment to take action. The message is then sent out to the appropriate muscle group to take action and to withdraw the hand.

A much more complicated scenario is that of a basketball player who receives a pass while racing toward the basket. Between him and the basket are the defenders of the opposite team. The offensive player must appraise the defenses and decides whether to take the shot, dribble, or pass off to a team mate, then to take the appropriate action. All of this is done while running at top speed. That is a very complicated set of choices, yet it is resolved in less than a second.

Carry the scenario a step farther. A surgeon in the course of an operation encounters severe bleeding in a very delicate and essential part of the body. He/she must instantly review his/her knowledge of the anatomy of the region, decide on the consequences of various actions, then carry out the proper course of action-all within seconds.

These illustrations point out the ability of the central nervous system to deal with information from the outside world. Imagine the complexity of the task for the brain to simultaneously process a continuous flow of information from all parts of the body as rapidly as the information is received. The power of this "super computer" is awesome, and far from being completely understood. Statements have often been made by knowledgeable physiologists, psychologists and educators that most of us use only a small percentage of the potential power of our brains during a lifetime.

THE ANATOMY OF THE NERVOUS SYSTEM

For the purposes of this book, which is a primer of medicine, not a real textbook of medicine, the discussion of the anatomy of the brain and the spinal cord to follow will be quite sketchy. Only the large picture will be presented. For the reader who wishes more complete information there are a number of excellent texts on neuro-anatomy available at any medical library.

THE SKULL AND THE MENINGES

In addition to being one of the most vital organs of the body the brain has the distinction of being the most fragile and delicate organ. Brain tissue has the consistency of gelatin, or of custard. Fortunately, the brain is encased in layers of very protective covering, the skull and the meninges.

The skull, discussed in detail in the chapter on the skeleton, is a hard bony shell that provides good protection against mild and moderate injuries. Within the shell of the skill are two layers of fibrous tissue that encase the brain and continue downward into the spinal canal as layers surrounding that fragile structure. Together they are called the Meninges. The outer layer, called the Dura Mater, is thick and tough and carries blood vessels that penetrate and enter the brain. The inner layer is very thin and cobweb-like, and makes contact with the brain tissue. It is called the Pia Mater. If the meninges become inflamed or infected the condition is called meningitis, a word that is probably familiar to most readers.

THE ANATOMY OF THE BRAIN

The brain is divided into two halves that are connected by a vast number of nerve fibers. Because the shape of the brain is roughly that of a sphere cut in half, and because the Greek name for the brain is Cerebrum, the two halves are called Cerebral hemispheres. The surface of the brain is deeply wrinkled with folds that add greatly to the surface area of the brain. Each hemisphere is divided into four lobes: the frontal, temporal, parietal, and occipital lobes, going from front to back.

The most superficial portion of the cerebrum, called the cerebral cortex, is gray in appearance because it is composed of nerve cells. That layer is called the gray matter of the brain. Those millions of nerve cells constitute the place where memory and association and the making of decisions take place. They are the heart of the computer. The deeper- lying cells are white in appearance because they are neurons, nerve fibers that have sheathes. They function as the wires, connecting the cells of the gray matter. The sheath material is called myelin, which is composed largely of fat and protein. The function of myelin sheathes is to insulate the nerve fibers, much as insulation is placed around electrical wires. Myelinated nerve fibers are also found outside of the spinal cord in the peripheral nerves.

Nerve fibers that are covered with myelin have a special quality conferred by the sheath: If they are severely damaged they can usually heal within the myelin covering and can grow to surprising length to end in their normal destination. Unmyelinated nerve tissue cannot heal or recover if damaged. Hence, a severe injury to the gray matter of the brain is likely to leave a permanent area of non-functional tissue. That becomes extremely important if a stroke or tumor destroys an area of gray matter.

The brain has been recognized as the center for thought and decision making since the early times of anatomy scholars. Areas of the brain were designated to have specific functions many years ago. However, only in the last half of the nineteenth century was it learned that the brain does not have pain sensors, and therefore that brain surgery could be performed with the patient awake and comfortable. That finding led to early experiments in which weak electrical stimuli were applied to various areas of the cerebral cortex, and the resultant effect charted. Thus the mapping of the brain areas began. With the availability of MRI imaging, and PET imaging, mapping of the brain is beginning to become an exact science, although still in its early days.

Lying deep within the brain is a structure called the thalamus, an important relay center that connects the various parts of the brain. Just below the thalamus is the hypothalamus that regulates the functions of the autonomic nervous system, the endocrine glands, and many somatic bodily functions. Those are primitive parts of the brain, meaning that those parts have been identified in the brains of more primitive animals. Their function is to manage the ongoing workings of the basic nonintellectual functioning of the brain.

The cerebellum is the portion of the brain that is located posteriorly and below the cerebral hemispheres. It consists of a median lobe and a pair of lateral lobes which are globular structures with wrinkled surfaces, resembling in size and shape a pair of walnuts. The nerve cells and fibers of the cerebellum are largely responsible for muscle coordination and the sense of balance and equilibrium.

The next part of the brain, extending posteriorly, and ending in the spinal cord is the hindbrain, or brain stem. This is developmentally the most primitive part of the brain, similar to that found in lower animals. The brain stem connects the cerebral hemispheres with the spinal cord and controls the basic vegetative functions of the body, such as breathing and heartbeat.

Extending directly outward from the brain stem are twelve important paired nerves that are called the cranial nerves. These nerves leave the brain stem through a series of openings in each side of the skull and go to the regions of the head and face. The first three of those paired nerves arise from the cerebrum. They carry the sense of smell, the sense of vision and the movements of the eyes. The next nine pairs of cranial nerves arise from the brain stem. They go to the head and face, providing sensation and the nerve supply to the nose, eyes, facial muscles, tongue, ears, throat, and to the heart, lungs, chest and abdomen.

The brain stem, a thick stalk of nerve fibers, exits the skull through an opening called the foramen magnum, and the nerve tissue then becomes the spinal cord.

Before going on to the spinal cord it seems appropriate to make some general comments about the brain at this point. The cerebral hemispheres determine the "handedness" of an individual. The left hemisphere is functionally dominant over the right hemisphere in a person who is right-handed. It is also slightly larger and heavier than the right hemisphere in right- handed people. The opposite is true in a person who is naturally left- handed. It is a generally accepted fact that in right-handed people the left hemisphere dominates over the right in intellectual activity, and the right hemisphere over the left in artistic behavior and capability.

The opposite is also true in people who are naturally left-handed. A stroke or major injury involving the left hemisphere is much more disabling to a right-handed person than if it would be in the right hemisphere, and the reverse is true for left-handed individuals. There is a slight difference in the brains of a female and a male. In addition to being slightly smaller on the average, because women are smaller than men on the average, the nerve tracts of the hypothalamus are larger and more complex in women than in men. This may correlate with the more active interests of women in endeavors involving "right brain capability." There is absolutely no evidence that the structure of the brain differs significantly in individuals of various racial origins or ethnic or religious preference.

THE SPINAL CORD

The spinal cord is the second part of the central nervous system. It extends from the base of the skull to the end of the lumbar spine. The spinal cord, as the brain, is composed of tissue that has almost no intrinsic strength of its own. Fortunately, it travels through its entire length within the protection of the vertebral column (the spine). Each vertebra in the spinal column has an opening in either side, called the foramina, through which spinal nerves exit and enter.

The spinal cord is also protected within the bony tunnel of the spine by the meninges, the membranes that encase the brain within the skull. The meninges carry the arteries and veins that supply blood to the spinal cord. They also serve as cushioning to protect the delicate tissue of the spinal cord against injury.

The spinal cord gives off a pair of nerve roots through the foramina at each vertebral level to the left and the right sides of the body. In general those nerve roots divide into many branches that supply the skin, muscles and organs at that level of the body. Sensory nerves from all the organs at each level of the spine enter through those foramina to make connections with other nerves that carry their messages to the brain.

There are seven vertebrae in the cervical (neck) region. The nerves from that region supply the organs located in the neck and chest and diaphragm.

There are twelve vertebrae in the thoracic segment of the spine. The nerves that leave and enter the spine at those levels supply the organs within the chest cavity, the chest wall, the upper back and the upper extremities, extending to the fingertips.

There are five vertebrae in the lumbar segment of the spine. The nerves that leave and enter the first and second lumbar vertebrae supply the organs within the abdominal cavity, and the abdominal wall. Below that level the spinal nerves from the third, fourth and fifth vertebral levels provide motor and sensory branches via nerve filaments called the cauda equina to the lowest organs of the pelvis and to the lower extremities.

THE PERIPHERAL NERVOUS SYSTEM

That is the name given to the very extensive system of nerves that stem from the nerve trunks that make connections with the spinal nerves at each level of the vertebral column. Functioning much like a two- way switchboard, those nerves extend to every organ of the body. There are many sub-connections and interconnections in this system. Those nerves that serve a sensory function, sending information to the brain remain separate from the motor nerves that carry commands from the brain to the muscles and organs of the body. There are sensory-motor reflex pathways that cause automatic response, such as the familiar knee-jerk, and many others which are much more complicated.

Peripheral nerves have myelin sheathes, similarly to the nerves that constitute the white matter of the brain All of the organs of the body that are under voluntary control are provided with motor and sensory nerves.

THE AUTONOMIC NERVOUS SYSTEM

This is the third component of the nervous systems of the body. It is composed of nerve elements from the central nervous system and from the peripheral nervous system. They meet in a series of connections called ganglia that are located on each side of the vertebral column throughout its length. There are two components to the autonomic nervous system: the sympathetic nervous system and the parasympathetic nervous system.

The sympathetic nervous system serves as the protector of the body against real or perceived danger. It carries messages to the medulla of the adrenal gland, telling it to secrete adrenaline and it tells the heart, the blood vessels throughout the body and the organs of respiration, digestion, urine formation and even the skin that it is time for flight or fight and to prepare for that state.

Unfortunately, as described in the chapter on the endocrine system, the sympathetic nervous system is also controlled in part by the brain. A state of sustained emotional stress or anxiety can result in severe over-activity of the sympathetic nervous system. That can cause high blood pressure, spasm of the arteries in many areas of the body and damage to the digestive system due to shunting of blood away from the gut to the muscles of flight or fight. Another effect of over-activity of the sympathetic nervous system is to cause the blood vessels within the skin to constrict, forcing the blood from the enormous network of vessels within the skin, and directing that blood into the skeletal muscles, the heart and the brain to enable the body to flee, or fight. This causes the skin of the hands and feet to become cold, which accounts for the expression "he has cold feet", referring to one's reluctance to enter into a given activity, or deal.

The parasympathetic nervous system has the opposite function to that of the sympathetic nervous system. It has been referred to as "the housekeeper of the body" because its main function is to cause relaxation of the process just described, as the result of the action of the sympathetic nervous system.

The nerve endings of both the sympathetic and parasympathetic systems act upon muscles that are different from the muscles of volition that operate our arms and legs and other muscles that are controlled consciously. The difference between those muscles will be discussed in detail in the chapter on the musculoskeletal system.

In the normal state of health the parasympathetic nervous system operates as a balancing force in opposition to the sympathetic system. That mechanism of checks and balances operates continuously and without conscious awareness or volitional control.

In the above description of the functioning of the nervous system there have been many references to the passage of nerve impulses from one nerve to another and from nerves to muscles. The implication is that this transmission is purely electrical, similarly to that in the electrical systems within our home. That is not the case. Neural transmission is far more complicated than that. The connections between one nerve and another and between nerves and muscles are by means of connectors called synapses. To add a bit more to the complication; the nerve endings are called axons and dendrites. At the terminal ends of synapses are microscopic glandular structures that produce and secrete chemical substances in microscopic amounts. The chief of those chemical Compounds are called acetylcholine and norepinephrine. The very small amount of electrical energy in a single nerve impulse causes the release of one of those neuro-transmitting compounds, resulting in stimulation of the synaptic end of the next nerve fiber and the passage of the nerve impulse from one nerve to another, or from nerve to muscle. Keeping in mind that neural transmissions occur in milliseconds, at many sites simultaneously throughout every second of our lives, this concept is mind-boggling.

This has been a very brief description of the anatomy and physiology of the nervous system. That system in its infinite detail is the subject of many extensive treatises, and the life work of a great many brilliant and dedicated scientists. I have tried merely to give the reader a brief working overview of the subject from which to go farther.

DISORDERS OF THE NERVOUS SYSTEM

Dementia

It is a commonly known fact that the lifespan in this country, as it has in most of the developed nations of the world, has increased significantly over the past half-century. This is chiefly due to better living conditions and better understanding of diseases and their treatment. That has enhanced the ability of medical science to prevent and treat illnesses that were previously considered fatal. Another important factor has been better education about nutrition and the avoidance of toxic substances. It is a sad fact, however, that the reduction of pollution in our environment and the improvement in the understanding of good nutrition of a large segment of the population has a long way to go.

As wonderful as extending the average age by fifteen to twenty years in the past century is, it has opened the door to the increase of the diseases of aging.

It is very evident that the body undergoes changes that are directly related to becoming older. Joints become stiff and arthritic, muscles become weak, the skin becomes wrinkled and speckled, and cardio-vascular diseases increase greatly. Another change that has become more prominent these days than it has been in the past is the occurrence of dementia.

Dementia can be defined in several ways: the loss of cognition, memory loss, inappropriate behavior, and a general loss of the ability to take care of oneself. Dementia, in most instances, is due to the loss of functioning cells in the gray matter of the cerebral cortex. The classic reason for that is a change in the arterial blood vessels that supply the gray matter. As in other parts of the body there is a tendency for atherosclerosis to occur in the cerebral blood supply. As the tiny arteries and arterioles become blocked the brain tissue becomes deprived of oxygen and nutrients, and as a result there is death of nerve cells.

The death of cells anywhere in the body as the result of deprivation of blood supply is called infarction. When the cells that die are in the gray matter of the brain and their death causes a change in mental capacity that condition is called "multi-infarction dementia."

That concept of the cause of dementia is certainly applicable in the present day, but over the past ten to fifteen years another cause for dementia has become increasingly evident. That is the syndrome called Alzheimer's disease, named after the physician who first described it.

The real cause of Alzheimer's disease is not known, but there is increasing evidence to suggest that it may be the result of some type of infection, or of some other disease process that destroys cells in the gray matter of the cerebral cortex. MRI studies have shown the consistent presence of some type of scarring in the brain cells of Alzheimer's patients that has been documented by microscopic examination of brain tissue in post-mortem examination of patients with the Alzheimer's syndrome, but no causative organism has ever been isolated.

Patients who are diagnosed as having the Alzheimer syndrome frequently tend to become combative, often having severe rages and assaulting their care-givers. They are also subject to severe musculoskeletal contractures, rendering them completely confined to bed because of inability to extend their limbs, with severe muscle atrophy.

Dementia can also be caused by brain injury, especially by repeated traumas. This can be chemical, as in the case of chronic alcohol abuse or repeated exposure to drug substances, or physical, as in the case of a prizefighter who has received too many blows to the head, causing small areas of bleeding, with resultant loss of brain cells. .

At the present time there is no known cure for dementia caused by any of the above brain disorders. Care should be focused on efforts to encourage the saving of remaining brain function by strategies to encourage cognition and memory. There is some value in using the medications that are now available for the treatment of the Alzheimer syndrome, although none of them have been shown to be curative and the confidence level of their effectiveness is becoming questionable. The physical condition of the patient should be maintained as much as possible by a regular exercise program.

INFECTIONS OF THE NERVOUS SYSTEM

Meningitis

Meningitis is the name given to infection involving the meninges, the membranes that surround, protect, and nourish the brain and the spinal cord. The most common cause of meningitis is bacterial infection that is either blood-borne from some other site of infection, or by direct extension from an adjacent area, such as the nasopharynx or the sinuses. The site of the infection is either in the meninges surrounding the brain or in those surrounding the spinal cord, although it is common for both to be involved by direct extension. The causative organism is most commonly a bacterium called "the Meningococcus", or the common Streptococcus. Other bacteria can be involved, depending on the source of the infection.

In the case of cerebral meningitis there is usually severe headache and fever as the initial presenting symptom and sign. As the infection extends to the spinal meninges the most common sign is pain caused by flexion of the neck, and marked restriction of motion of the neck.

Meningitis originating in the spinal cord is not as common as cerebrospinal meningitis, although it can occur as the result of bacterial infection of the lower spinal cord or adjacent structures.

If not treated promptly and properly, meningitis can cause severe and permanent damage to the central nervous system. In most of those infections, however, the infecting organism is sensitive to the available antibiotics. There is truly a danger that most currently used antibiotics will become ineffective for the treatment of such diseases due to their futile over-use in treating common virus-caused infections.

It is not uncommon to have permanent after-effects in the form of partial loss of hearing, or of some other of the senses.

Aseptic Meningitis

Aseptic meningitis is a different form of meningitis that is not due to bacterial infection. There is no single specific cause, but viral infections and auto-immune reactions are listed as possible causes. The typical symptoms of meningitis are not characteristically seen, but fever, headache, stiffening of the neck and back can be present. This disorder is also seen as a manifestation of a generalized acute auto-immune demyelinating disorder bearing the name of Guillan-Barre syndrome.

Any form of meningitis is a serious disease, warranting hospital care and the services of a competent neurologist.

Encephalitis

Encephalitis is the name given to inflammation of the cells of the brain. The most common cause is acute viral infection. That can occur either as a complication of a common viral infection, such as measles, mumps or chickenpox, or as a complication of certain insect stings in which a virus is injected into the human system. At the time of this writing there is much concern over certain species of mosquitoes recently introduced into this country that are vectors of West Nile disease that includes acute encephalitis in its manifestations.

Encephalitis, being a non-bacterial infection; poses a serious problem in treatment as there is no antibiotic capable of affecting viral infections. If the causative virus is in the Herpes Simplex family there is better susceptibility to antiviral medications. In some cases there is severe residual brain damage. That is especially true in the case of infected infants and young children. In the case of severe epidemic viral encephalitis death of the patient is not unusual.

There is another form of viral infection that, fortunately, has been largely eradicated in the world. That is Acute Poliomyelitis, commonly called "Polio." That virus causes infection of the spinal cord, referred to as "myelitis." In past years poliomyelitis was responsible for many deaths and permanent crippling states. The widespread use of polio vaccines has reduced the incidence of that disease significantly, but it still lurks in the background as a possible source of future epidemics.

Stroke

Stroke is a very frequently seen disorder of the nervous system. The Doctor Speak name for stroke is "Cerebral Vascular Accident", usually abbreviated to CVA. That term specifically defines stroke as an interruption of the blood supply to a part of the brain, either by thrombosis or by hemorrhage. The most common type of stroke is the formation of a clot, (thrombus) within a cerebral artery, most commonly because of atheromatous plaque rupture, as was described in the discussion of a coronary heart attack. That results in the loss of the blood supply to a part of the brain. In most cases the area of loss is small, frequently unnoticed. However, if the thrombus is within a major artery the area of brain deprived of blood supply can be very large. Depending upon the area of the brain affected and the size of the blood vessel that is involved the severity can vary from no noted effect to a minor behavioral change or to major loss of function or to death.

The second and much less common cause of stroke is hemorrhage within the brain. That is most often due to high blood pressure, causing an artery to rupture and to bleed into the delicate brain tissue. Another cause of bleeding into the brain is rupture of an artery due to aneurysm, which is a weakness of the wall of an artery, usually congenital (present from birth). With the passage of time and often enhanced by high blood pressure, the weak area becomes distended, the wall of the artery becomes thin and eventually ruptures.

The clinical appearance of stroke from either thrombosis or hemorrhage is, in most cases the same. There may be a change in the patient's appearance, such as weakness of an extremity or sagging of the facial muscles on one side. The speech may suddenly become slurred or absent. There may be loss of consciousness, dizziness, nausea, or some other abrupt behavioral change. Headache is not always present in a stroke scenario. Any of those changes could signal the early signs of stroke. That person should be hospitalized immediately, by paramedic ambulance, for close observation and early treatment.

In the hospital emergency room the patient should be examined at once as a potential major emergency. In most cases a CT scan will be the first procedure done. In the event that it shows evidence of bleeding into the brain it indicates that the cause is a hemorrhage, possibly requiring an immediate neurosurgical operation. If there is no evidence of bleeding the likelihood of a thrombosis increases. In either case, emergency care should be instituted at once, best given by a neurologist or a neurosurgeon; if possible, although today's E.R. physicians are usually well trained in the emergency treatment of cerebral thrombosis.

With the techniques that are available at this time and provided that proper emergency care is instituted promptly, there is a good likelihood that the patient will do well if the cause of the stroke is thrombosis. Cerebral hemorrhage carries a poorer prognosis if the bleeding is deeply within the substance of the brain. Superficial bleeding in the region of the meninges can usually be greatly relieved by prompt surgical intervention.

Transient Ischemic Attack

That is the name given to a event in which there is a temporary interruption of the blood supply to an area of the brain. The Doctor Speak shorthand term for it is "T.I.A." It is most likely caused by a temporary spasm of an artery within the brain. The signs and symptoms may mimic those of a stroke, being a visible change, such as a loss of muscle control in a localized part of the body or a behavioral change, such as the slurring of speech or total loss of ability to speak or even loss of consciousness. The factor that differentiates a T.I.A. from a stroke is the transient nature of the episode. In can last from minutes to hours, but if it resolves spontaneously it is by definition not a stroke. In most cases the individual appears to be totally normal following a T.I.A. That person, however, should have a follow-up neurologic examination to evaluate the cerebral circulation. Most commonly a duplex scan of the carotid arteries is included in that examination to rule out atherosclerotic narrowing. There is a statistically greater likelihood of stroke in individuals who have had a T.I.A. In most cases no specific treatment is advised, other than taking a baby aspirin daily to reduce the likelihood of thrombus formation.

Seizure States

This is another type of disorder of the brain, formerly called epilepsy. That term is no longer used in medical parlance.

There are two types of seizures that are most commonly seen. The most common is referred to as a general seizure. In the old terminology it was called a "grand mal seizure." It usually begins as jerking and thrashing movements of the extremities and the entire body, often accompanied by groaning sounds and cries. The first sign is often a twitching movement of small muscle groups. The twitching then extends to large muscle groups and often to the entire body. The patient has no evidence of conscious awareness of what is going on. The episodes can last only moments or can go on for many minutes. During that time there may be severe disturbance of breathing, and, in fact, some danger of asphyxia because the tongue can fall into the airway and prevent breathing, or there can be spasm of the muscles of the larynx, obstructing the airway. Afterward, the patient has complete amnesia for the entire episode.

The cause of general seizures is an uncontrolled random electrical activity of neurons within the motor area of the brain. In most cases the cause of that phenomenon is unknown. In some cases the source of the stimulation of those motor neurons can be identified as scar tissue caused by some earlier injury to the brain. That scar tissue acts as a local irritant stimulating the adjacent normal brain tissue. The former is referred to in medical parlance as an "idiopathic seizure", meaning "cause unknown." The latter is called a "Jacksonian seizure", after the physician who first described that type of seizure.

General seizures most often are first seen in the age range of twenty to thirty, and can continue episodically for the rest of a person's life, although they are not rare in children and youngsters under twenty.

Another type of seizure state occurs most commonly in school age children, and often continues into the twenties, then, in many cases subsides. That kind of seizure is called "absence seizure." In the old terminology it was called "petit mal epilepsy." A good example of absence seizure is that which might occur while a child is in class. The patient becomes quite still, usually sitting upright, with eyes open. That state can remain for many minutes then subsides spontaneously. The patient has absolutely no awareness that the event was occurring, and has amnesia for the period of time that was involved. There is no abnormal motor behavior in the classic absence seizure. The patient can usually resume normal activity after the seizure.

There are other classifications of seizure states, but the ones described are the most commonly seen types.

Seizure states of all types can most often be managed with medication taken orally. In some cases it is essential for the medication to be taken for life. In the case of a first episode seizure of any kind it is common practice to treat the patient with medication for six months, during which time operating a vehicle or dangerous equipment is forbidden. After six months the medication can be stopped for a period of observation. If no seizure occurs within a year the patient is merely observed with no further medication and driving can be resumed. If seizures do recur after the medication is stopped it is customary to resume the medication for another six months, and then stop for another period of observation. If seizures recur the patient is usually asked to remain on medication for life.

Tremor States

The term "tremor" refers to uncontrollable rapid shaking movements of muscle groups in various parts of the body. Tremor states are caused by disease processes in the motor area of the brain, except for the trembling seen in a person whose thyroid gland is hyperactive, causing over-stimulation of the nervous system, as well as that of the cardiovascular system and other parts of the body.

There are two general types of tremors that are caused by brain dysfunction: Parkinsonian, the name derived from the physician who first described the condition and non-Parkinsonian tremors. The latter will be described first.

Non-Parkinsonian tremors are generally referred to as "benign essential tremors." Those tremors often begin with rapid shaking of the head and neck and then extend to the hands, arms and then to the lower extremities in some cases, although most commonly the trembling is confined to the head and neck. Those tremors rarely become disabling and are quite resistant to treatment. They usually begin in the forties or later and usually last for life.

Parkinsonian tremors are actually manifestations of a disease that involves the motor center of the brain and most often becomes progressively more severe with the passage of time. The first manifestation is usually in one or both hands, involving the thumb and index finger. It is described as "a pill-rolling movement", because in the early days of medicine pharmacists made their own pills and shaped them by rolling the material between their thumb and index finger.

Parkinson's disease usually begins in the late forties or fifties and becomes progressively more severe with the passage of time as more motor neurons become diseased. A common manifestation of the disease is progressive rigidity and difficulties of gait because the nerves supplying the opposing muscles of the legs send false and simultaneous messages to the legs, causing stiffness, weakness, and a shuffling gait. As Parkinson's disease progresses there is involvement of the muscles of the voice and of respiration in severe cases. The latter is the leading cause of death from that disease.

Parkinson's disease can be treated with oral medications which in most cases are adequate to control the disease for the life of the patient. In the severe form, as the disease progresses medications fail to control its progress. Brain surgery has been the topic of discussion among physicians for many years, but has generally failed to control the severe manifestations that lead to major disability and death. There is a recent resurgence of interest in the surgical treatment of Parkinson's disease. The use of stem cells to be implanted surgically into the diseased motor area of the brain is currently being advocated as a means of replacing the damaged brain cells that cause the disorder. It is still early days, but help may be on the way.

There are other types of tremors that are specifically the result of small strokes and specific brain injuries but those described above are the most commonly seen tremor states.

Multiple Sclerosis

This is a disease of the central nervous system, involving myelinated nerve fibers, both motor and sensory. It is classed as an "auto-immune disease". The cause of that entire class of disease is not known. Because of this disease process the myelin sheathes that cover and insulate some nerves are damaged and destroyed. This causes loss of sensory function in the affected nerve pathways and loss of motor function in the muscles innervated by the affected nerves.

The onset of multiple sclerosis is usually in the forties or fifties in most instances. Women are more frequently affected than are men. The disease has intermittent exacerbations during which symptoms appear or worsen and remissions in which the symptoms do not progress, but remain stable. A period of exacerbation can last from days to months and remissions cal last for years with no apparent evidence of new disease.

The most frequently seen initial signs of multiple sclerosis involve weakness of muscle groups, most frequently in a leg, or loss of equilibrium and dizziness because of involvement of the nerves of the cerebellum. However, a sudden change in function of any part of the body should be considered as a possible first sign of this disease. Because the myelin sheathes are destroyed by the disease process there is usually no recovery of the affected nerve. Speech, hearing, and vision can be affected also. Multiple sclerosis does not affect intellectual function, which resides in the gray matter which is composed of unmyelinated nerves of the cerebral cortex.

Multiple sclerosis is usually affected adversely by heat. Therefore it is advisable for those patients to avoid hot baths and hot weather. There is no specific medication to remedy this disease. A vigorous program of exercise is strongly recommended. Active participation in intellectual pursuits and group activities is a great help. The motto in this disease, as it is in many chronic illnesses is "push back, and do not give in to the disease."

There are many other diseases, some of which are familiar to the reader, such as "Lou Gehrig's disease", the proper name of which is amyotrophic lateral sclerosis, or ALS, but they are far less common and It would serve no purpose to catalog those in this book. Excellent textbooks of neurology are easily available to those who would pursue the subject.

The nervous system suffers greatly in other systemic diseases such as diabetes or hypothyroidism or alcoholism. Because of the intrinsic sensitivity of the brain and other elements of the nervous system those neurologic manifestations are viewed as side-effects of the primary disorder.

Brain Tumors

Headache is almost never a sign of a cancer or tumor of the brain. Cancer of the brain is not uncommon. It can occur as a primary disease, originating within the brain. It is more common, however, for malignant tumors of the brain to be metastatic, originating in other organs of the body. In each case the cancer is most often diagnosed because of some failure of brain function producing neurological changes elsewhere in the body.

There are also many benign tumors that originate in the brain. Even though they are not classed as cancer, benign tumors can damage the brain tissue by the very fact of their enlargement causing pressure on the brain tissue against the hard case of the skull. The first symptoms and signs of benign tumors of the brain, as in the case of cancers of the brain, are most often the dysfunction of some remote part of the body that is affected by the part of the brain that is damaged by the tumor.

Neurosurgical procedures are commonly done for the treatment of benign tumors of the brain. Whatever surgical procedure is done on whatever part of the brain, it must be kept in mind that the brain tissue is very fragile and the resultant ill-effects of the surgery may be unpredictable.

It would not be helpful to attempt to give a specific description of the various known types of benign and malignant tumors of the brain or other parts of the nervous system in this book. The first and most important diagnostic signs and symptoms are, in the great majority of cases, failure or dysfunction of some part of the body that is secondarily affected by the tumor. Making the diagnosis and designing the treatment can be extremely complicated. In all cases it is ultimately necessary to have consultation with a neurologist or neurosurgeon.

Head Injuries

Brain tissue has no intrinsic strength. Especially in children, whose heads are heavier proportionately than the rest of their bodied; a fall that seems trivial can result in the brain moving within the skull and striking the hard bone of the skull. This also applies to adults. Any bump that is hard enough to cause even momentary loss of consciousness is called a cerebral concussion. Any bruise of the brain is called a cerebral contusion. Some concussions cause headaches. That is called a post-concussion headache. Some post-concussion headaches can last for days or weeks. If no other symptoms appear, such headaches warrant observation only.

Any head injury resulting in loss of consciousness deserves very careful examination. C.T. scan of the head is a procedure that will, in most cases, reveal any evidence of bleeding within the skull as the result of injury. C.T. scanning should therefore be done. In the event of intracranial bleeding or if the patient remains comatose a neurosurgical consultation should be obtained immediately. A small monitoring device can be placed within the skull to measure intra-cranial pressure. If the pressure within the skull increases as the result of slow bleeding from the injury some sort of surgical procedure can be done immediately to protect the brain from further damage.

On the other side of the coin is the instance in which a severe head injury results in a fracture of the skull, demonstrated on C.T. scan, or X-ray. If no evidence of intra-cranial bleeding is seen the decision is usually made to do nothing other than to observe the patient. The rationale for this is the same as if a Stradivarius violin is carried inside a wooden case, and is dropped. If the case breaks, but the violin is undamaged, no great harm has been done. However, any injury in which the skull is fractured must be monitored very carefully.

Headache

Every headache is serious and important to the patient. Headaches come in all sizes and shapes. They can be squeezing, stabbing, pulsating, or just there. They can be made worse by bright light and relieved by darkness, made worse by moving the head or bending over and relieved by lying still. Some headaches can be relieved by aspirin or Tylenol, ice packs and lying still in a dark room and others require strong medicine.

There is good news and bad news about headache. The good news is that headache is only rarely caused by a brain tumor, and very rarely by a brain cancer. Most of the mass of brain tissue does not have any pain receptors and so is not capable of causing headache.

The area of the meninges immediately within the skull, however, is richly supplied with pain-sensory nerves. After a fall or other head injury severe headache may be a sign of intracranial bleeding or swelling and must be monitored very carefully.

The vast majority of headaches are due to some form of migraine. Although migraine is very common, the cause and pathophysiology (what events occur within the brain) remains obscure. There is good evidence that dilation of intra-cranial blood vessels occurs, but the cause of that is not known. The symptoms of migraine and the pattern of the headache vary greatly. In some cases there is nausea and vomiting. Sometimes there is distortion of vision. There is no clear and fixed pattern of symptoms. Migraine is sometimes triggered by a state of tension, but that is not always the case. Allergy is often mentioned as a cause of migraine, but only in some cases. Medications are sometimes very effective in relieving the pain of migraine headaches but the headache can be very persistent. A medical consultation should be obtained if migraine headaches are severe and persistent.

Arthritis in the cervical spine can trigger headaches. Some headaches are a sign of high blood pressure, or an abnormal blood vessel within the cranium, or a tumor or blood clot that could and should be treated. Headaches that occur at times of severe anxiety or stress are often related to sustained muscle tension in the muscles of the back of the neck, and are usually felt in the occipital region of the head (in the very back of the head). They are usually referred to as "tension headaches." If such headaches persist they should be investigated to rule out a more serious cause.

My best advice is to not wait. If you are concerned, see your doctor. It could set your mind at ease and possibly avert serious trouble.

Chapter Eight
THE ORGANS OF SPECIAL SENSES

THE EYES—THE SENSE OF VISION
THE EARS—SENSES OF HEARING AND EQUILIBRIUM
THE SENSES OF TOUCH AND PAIN
THE SENSE OF TASTE
THE SENSE OF SMELL

THE EYES—SENSE OF VISION

In the previous chapters we have taken an anatomical and physiological tour of each system under discussion and have discovered amazing complexity in each of those. The eyes are certainly no exception to that rule. The eyes have the capability of converting physical energy in the form of light waves into chemical energy, then to electrical energy in the form of nerve impulses to the brain. This all happens instantaneously and continuously throughout a lifetime. That is impressive, even in comparison to the mysteries of the digital camera.

Now we will embark on our anatomical tour of the eye. As in the earlier sections of the book we will discuss the anatomy, physiology and biochemistry of each part of the eye. In addition, where it is applicable we will review the most common disorders that affect each part of the eye.

THE ANATOMY AND PHYSIOLOGY OF THE EYES

The Eyelids

The outermost part of the eye is the eyelid. The externally presenting part of the id is made of soft skin that is folded horizontally, allowing the eyelid to retract when the eye is widely open and to stretch enough to cover the bulb of the eye when the lid is closed. Immediately behind the skin is a layer of thick, tough fiber called the tarsal layer. That layer gives the skin of the lid a backing that allows it to open and close and to remain in either of those positions. The opening and closing of the eyelids is powered by small muscles that originate in the frontal and facial bones of the skull, and ligaments that end in the tarsal region of the lids. The nerve supply is a combination of autonomic and voluntary control. The autonomic nerves cause the lids to close involuntarily if the eye is touched, or irritated by a foreign body or substance. The voluntary nerves command normal opening and closing of the lids.

The Conjunctiva

Immediately behind the tarsal layer is the third layer of the eyelid that is called the conjunctival layer, or the conjunctiva. This is a thin, transparent membrane that is very complex in construction. It contains blood vessels and nerves from the voluntary and autonomic nervous systems. The conjunctiva covers the lid completely. It then folds onto the surface of the eyeball. The part that is attached to the lid is called the palpebral conjunctiva, referring to the lid as the palpebrum. That part of the conjunctiva that covers the eyeball is called the bulbar conjunctiva. At the edges of the eyelids are the lashes that serve as screens to keep large objects, such as insects, from touching the eyeball. At the base of each lash are an oil gland and a hair follicle that serves to lubricate and nourish the eyelash. If the hair follicle becomes infected there is a swelling at the base of the lash with redness of the surrounding skin. That condition is called a stye (hordeolum). In the center of the lid, located between the tarsal layer and the conjunctival layer are large glandular structures called Meibomian glands. They manufacture and secrete a lubricating fluid that bathes the eyes continuously.

If a Meibomian gland becomes infected because of some obstruction of the outflow of its fluid the eyelid becomes red and swollen, then, after a few days the infected gland swells to the point that it can be seen and felt through the skin of the eyelid. The name given to that disorder is chalazion. While most styes are easily treated in the office of your family doctor, chalazions usually require the services of an ophthalmologist.

The tear glands (lacrimal glands) are located high in the upper outer corner of each eyelid. They are about the size and shape of a small almond. The tears then wash across the surface of the conjunctiva and are drained into the fold of the lower lid. They are then conducted to the tear sac, a small mound of pink-red tissue located in the medial corner of each eye. From the tear sac they enter the tear duct that is the entrance to the nasolacrymal duct that drains the tears into the passages of the nose.

The nerve supply of the conjunctival layer of the eye is partly sensory, providing the information that something is “in the eye”, potentially injurious to the eye, and partly from motor nerves under control of the autonomic nervous system The flow of tears from the lacrimal glands is an effort to wash out any foreign body present on the conjunctival surface or, of course, a response to an emotional state. In either case the flow is triggered by the autonomic nervous system.

Any infection or injury of the bulbar or palpebral conjunctiva causes dilation of the small blood vessels, creating a "bloodshot" appearance to the eye. That usually remains until the injury subsides. The presence of the "bloodshot" dilated vessels brings to the conjunctival capillaries an extra supply of blood cells to increase resistance to infection.

The Sclera and Cornea

The layer of the eye just below the conjunctiva is called the sclera. That is a tough thick white layer of tissue that we call "the white of the eye." The sclera envelops most of the eye and is responsible for maintaining the globe-like shape of the eyeball.

The sclera covers the eyeball with the exception of a round opening in the center of the eye. That opening is covered by another structure called the cornea. The cornea is a thick transparent membrane of cells that connects at its outer margin with the sclera. Through the transparent cornea the black opening of the pupil is seen. The bulbar conjunctiva that covers the sclera ends at the margin of the cornea and does not cover the cornea. A healthy cornea allows full transmission of light waves through the pupil without distortion.

The Iris and The Pupil

The size of the pupillary opening is controlled by a unique structure called the iris of the eye. The iris is suspended between the cornea anteriorly and the lens posteriorly. It consists of two layers of plates of pigmented epithelial cells arranged in a radial manner. The pigment in the cells confers the color to the eye, and is present in all people except albinos, whose bodies lack all pigment. The optical density of the iris is such that only minimal light can pass through it. There is only one pigment for all eyes. It is called melanin pigment. The degree of concentration of the melanin causes variation in the color of individual eyes from pale blue to very dark brown.

The pigmented plates of cells of the iris extend from the inner edge of the pupil to the outer margin of the iris. At its outer margins the iris is connected to two layers of muscles. There is a strong layer that pulls in a radial direction, opening the iris, and a weaker layer of muscle arranged circumferentially that closes the iris. When wide open the iris causes the pupil to dilate, admitting more light. When the muscles of the iris relax and the opening of the pupil is smaller less light is admitted to the inner eye.

The nerve supply that controls the muscles of the iris is completely autonomic, not under purposeful control of the individual. It is a reflex action, controlled by the amount of light that enters the eye. That reflex action protects the light- sensitive structures at the back of the eye from injury due to overly strong light and also, when widely dilated in very low light, admits a maximum of light to enhance vision.

There is another element of control of the muscles of the iris that also is part of the autonomic nervous system. When an individual is highly stressed as the result of perceived or actual danger, or in any agitated state, the sympathetic nervous system comes into action, sending a message to the muscles of the iris to contract; thereby widening the pupil to allow maximal light to reach the retinal structures at the back of the eye. When that "emergency" state passes the parasympathetic nerves signal the muscles of the iris to relax, allowing the size of the pupil to become smaller.

The Lens

Immediately behind the iris is the lens of the eye. The lens is round in frontal profile, and oval shaped in lateral profile. It is constructed of a thick outer capsule that is completely clear and transparent and an inner structure of transparent plates of epithelial cells. At the margins of the lens are the attachments of strong ligaments that connect with strong muscles.

Until this point we have been discussing the eye as a structure that is remarkably similar to the cameras that we have known. The lid is the outer cover; the cornea is the inner glass protector of the lens. The iris is similar to the F-stop opening in regulating the amount of light that enters the camera. When we come to the lens and from that point on, the eye differs greatly from old cameras we have known with fixed lenses. Here the eye resembles the modern "auto-focus lens" cameras.

To enable the eye to focus on distant objects the lens must be as flat as possible, allowing the light rays to pass in parallel lines to the retina so that the largest possible image is focused upon the retina. In order to see objects that are very close or to read fine print, or to see any small object closely the lens must assume a more rounded shape. A rounded lens bends the incoming rays of light, focusing them for the desired viewing on the most sensitive part of the retina. The eye does that by means of the strong musculo-ligamentous bands that are attached to the lens. By pulling from both sides the contour of the lens is flattened to obtain the desired flat shape for distance vision. When the muscles are relaxed the lens is allowed to assume its rounded shape to facilitate near vision. The tension of those muscles is under the direction of voluntary control from the cerebral cortex. It is actually a learned behavior, beginning very early in the life of an infant and is not an autonomic or automatic action.

The part of the eye that we have been discussing, lying between the cornea and the lens is known as the anterior chamber of the eye. It is filled with a clear fluid called the aqueous, or in the old literature, the "aqueous humor." Going deeper into the eye, behind the lens, we encounter the posterior chamber of the eye. We will now move into that area.

The Posterior Chamber and Retina

When light rays pass through the lens they enter the posterior camber of the eye, also referred to as the vitreous body of the eye. It is a spacious area, filled with a thick transparent fluid called the vitreous. The light rays pass to the very back of the eye where they encounter the retina.

The retina is a curved sheet of tissue consisting of several layers of cells conforming to the curvature of the back of the eye. It is the counterpart of the film in a camera. The retina contains two types of light-sensitive structures called the cones and the rods. Those structures are spread out across the retina in a highly organized manner. The cones are capable of very fine discrimination of small images and close objects. They are concentrated in an area of the retina called the macula. The macula is located in the area of the retina at the point where incoming light rays are most directly focused by the lens.

The rods are located in a wide area surrounding the macula, least concentrated in the macula and extending to the periphery of the retina. They are capable of low-light discrimination and they enable peripheral vision. They are most effective in night vision, where the cones do not function well.

It is at this point that we discuss the most amazing properties of the eyes. Located in the base of each of those millions of cones and rods is a chemical receptor and a tiny nerve fiber. The chemical receptor receives a minute amount of physical energy from the incoming light waves that strike that particular cone or rod. That tiny amount of energy causes a chemical reaction to occur, in which a chemical compound called adenosine triphosphate, ATP for short, breaks down into adenosine diphosphate, ADP, releasing a small amount of electrical energy. That amount of electrical energy stimulates the tiny nerve fiber that then carries an electrical impulse to the head of the optic nerve, located at the posterior part of the retina.

The optic nerve gathers information instantly from millions of cone and rods and transmits it instantly to the visual cortex of the brain. The brain, meanwhile, receives information from the opposite eye via the same type of system. That information is instantly sent on to the memory and association centers of the brain and there translated from millions of bits of information, instantly, into a message of what the eyes have seen.

All of this goes on during every waking moment of a lifetime.

Immediately behind the layer of cones and rods is a very complex layer of blood vessels that provide circulation for the photosensitive layer, acting as a basement structure for the cones and rods. The blood vessels in that area are very commonly a source of medical problems, as we will see in the next part of this chapter.

Behind that layer and lying adjacent to the back of the eye is a dense layer of pigment called the choroid coat. That material corresponds to the thick black layer of light-absorbing material placed into the back of a camera.

The rear wall of the eyeball is the extension of the material called the sclera that we saw earlier as "the white of the eye." That thick, tough layer has openings through which pass the optic nerve to go to the brain and the arteries and veins that supply the eye.

COMMON DISORDERS OF THE EYE

STRABISMUS

The movements of the eye are precisely controlled by a set of muscles that originate at points in the bony orbits of the skull and attach to the bulb of the eye in such a way that they provide a very wide range of motion. Those muscles are controlled by messages from the brain with great precision.

Strabismus, "crossed eyes", is a congenital condition. It is due to improper location of the attachments of the muscles that control the positioning and movements of the eye. Strabismus usually occurs in one eye only but sometimes involves both eyes. The child usually realizes very early in life that only one eye is seeing properly and abandons the effort to use the information from the deviated eye.

The brain then accommodates to that disorder by ignoring messages from the affected eye and accepting messages only from the "good eye", even though the eye that deviates is usually optically perfect.

Strabismus can most often be corrected by a surgical operation in which the misplaced attachment of the eye muscle is replaced in its proper location. Strabismus should be corrected as early as possible in the first few years of the child's life before the brain has fixated on accepting messages only from one eye. If the surgery is delayed too long that person may go through life without true binocular vision and with two normally-functioning eyes that see independently of each other. That can affect depth perception quite seriously, but the individual usually adapts well to having one eye dominate the vision.

DISORDERS OF THE EYELIDS

The outer layer of skin of the lids is subject to all the problems of skin anywhere in the body, including injuries and growths that can be benign or malignant. Any growth on an eyelid should be seen by a physician and if necessary, be removed with care to avoid permanent deformity of the lid.

A very common condition of the eyelids is stretching and folding of the skin. In most cases the problem is only cosmetic, but as such is very important to the bearer. In a relatively small percentage of cases the excess lid tissue prevents proper opening of the lid, and must be corrected.

There is a neurological disorder called myasthenia gravis. It will be discussed in the chapter on the muscles. In that condition the muscles of the eyelids are severely weakened and unable to open or close the lids completely. Myasthenia gravis can be treated medically with good results in most cases.

DISORDERS OF THE CONJUNCTIVA

The innermost lining of the eyelid and the outermost covering of the bulb is the thin, transparent membrane called the conjunctiva. If a foreign body, such as a speck of sand or dust enters the eye there is immediate pain in the eye and dilation of the conjunctival blood vessels to cause a "bloodshot eye." Tears flow, and the end result is usually that the foreign body is washed away. If that does not occur it is often necessary to get medical help to remove the foreign body. The same occurs in the event of the splashing of an irritating liquid into the eye. The result is chemical injury, or chemical conjunctivitis. That condition must be attended to immediately to prevent permanent damage to the eye. As a general rule the affected eye should be irrigated copiously with water until professional help can be obtained.

Another serious problem is infection of the conjunctiva. That is usually by viral or bacterial organisms that come in contact with the conjunctiva, and is referred to as infectious conjunctivitis. A very common form of that infection is called "pink eye", in common terms. It is frequently seen in epidemic form in young school children. It is not unusual for many children in the same class to become infected through contact from child-to- child. It is in most cases a mild self-limiting disease, but should be seen by a physician.

DISORDERS OF THE CORNEA

The cornea is a very important part of the optical system of the eye. It is transparent and clear and rounded to be an integral part of the mechanism of focusing incoming waves of light as they enter the eye. Because of its exposed position, being in the very front of the eye, protected only by the eyelids and not having the protection of the conjunctiva, it is subject to serious injuries and diseases that can affect the function of the entire eye.

The problem most often affecting the cornea is physical or chemical injury. A particle thrown off by a grinding wheel or from any kind of tool that strikes the eye has a good chance of striking the cornea. It could result in a severe abrasion or laceration or even penetration of the cornea. The same applies to liquids that chance to splash into the eye. Depending on the severity of the injury and the quality of care given the end result could be permanent scarring of the cornea or no demonstrable residual injury. Severe scarring can affect the vision from that eye permanently. Infections that attack the cornea can also produce severe permanent scarring that can render that eye blind. The most common cause of blindness in the world is an infection called trachoma. That disease is prevalent in Africa and in underdeveloped countries. It is due to a bacterial infection of the cornea that causes severe scarring. Trachoma is curable with antibiotics applied to the eye and taken internally, but that treatment is often unavailable.

One of the most serious causes of corneal disease in our society is the virus of herpes zoster, (shingles). The infecting virus, traveling through a branch of a nerve supplying the eye can attack the cornea, causing severe scarring. Herpes infection of the cornea is a medical emergency, requiring expert and immediate care. Unless such an infection is treated promptly and properly the end result can be severe permanent scarring of the cornea. Such injuries sometimes require removal of the damaged cornea and transplantation of a donor cornea, a sometimes-hazardous procedure because of failure of the transplanted cornea to "take."

The other serious problem affecting the cornea is myopia, a congenital deformity of the cornea in which the curvature is excessive, resulting in abnormal bending of the incoming waves of light before they encounter the lens. That condition is usually detected early in life and can be corrected with eyeglasses, contact lenses, and sometimes with radial keratotomy surgery. That is a technique in which radial cuts are made in the cornea, causing it to flatten somewhat. That can reduce the excessive bending of incoming light rays. In recent years radial keratotomy has been performed using laser instruments. That has simplified the procedure. At the time of this writing there remains some difference of opinion as to the lasting value or radial keratotomy.

Another common congenital disorder of the cornea is astigmatism, which is a state of uneven curvature of the cornea. If not corrected, the cornea bends the incoming rays of light unevenly, delivering a distorted image to the lens and retina. In most cases this can be corrected with eyeglasses.

DISORDERS OF THE IRIS

The iris is subject to a serious inflammatory disorder called iritis. Iritis is classed as an auto-immune disorder.

The eye appears to be inflamed and vision is distorted. It is essential that proper medical care be given promptly to prevent permanent distortion of the iris. The treatment most commonly given is the use of corticosteroid medication applied topically and by mouth. The outcome of iritis is not always successful, resulting in permanent distortion of the iris, and reduced vision in the affected eye.

Serious physical trauma to the eye can damage the iris. In most cases that injury can be corrected by good surgical repair.

DISORDERS OF THE LENS

Hyperopia is a congenital disorder in which the lens is incapable of focusing on distant objects. Eyeglasses and contact lenses can usually correct that condition.

Presbyopia is the condition of inability to focus on small or near objects. That condition commonly occurs as a result of the aging process. Because of progressive stiffening due to aging the lens becomes unable to bend the incoming light waves sufficiently to focus on the retina. This condition can usually be corrected by the use of glasses.

Cataract

Cataract is among the most common causes of blindness in the world. The incidence is highest in underdeveloped nations. In the United States it is most commonly seen in the aged but it is also seen in young individuals. The basic underlying process is a change in the material within the capsule of the lens that causes it to become opaque and unable to transmit the light rays to the retina. The cause of that change is not clearly understood. In young individuals there is often a history of radiation of the lens with high-intensity light rays. In older people the cause is probably cumulative injury from light ray exposure. Certain illnesses such as diabetes increase the susceptibility to cataract formation. There is quite probably a congenital predisposition to cataract. The modern treatment for cataract is the removal of the diseased lens and replacement with an artificial lens in the same procedure. There is a very high success rate with that treatment.

DISORDERS OF THE RETINA

In our anatomical tour the retina was described in considerable detail. The part of the retina that is located at the approximate center of converging incoming light rays is called the fovea of the retina, and is also called the "macula" of the retina.

Immediately posterior to the layer of cones and rods is a network of nerve fibers that receive messages from the cones and rods, and a network of arteries and veins that service the photosensitive part of the retina. It is in that vascular portion of the retina that most retinal problems occur. The arteries and veins in that area are very small, but they can be seen very clearly through an optical instrument called an ophthalmoscope that is the standard equipment of most physicians. A medical doctor who treats the entire eye is called an ophthalmologist. Some ophthalmologists are specially trained to treat disorders of the retina. They are called retinologists. The retinal area and most specifically the vitreous and neuro-vascular part of the retina is where they spend most of their working days.

The above two paragraphs are introductions to the problems of that most complicated part of the eye, the retina.

Retinal Detachment

That is a condition in which the retinal layers become separated from the backing layer, the choroid. It occurs most commonly in people who are severely myopic, and following cataract surgery. In some cases there is tearing of the retinal layer with partial detachment, and in other instances the entire retinal layer separates from its backing. The symptoms are a sudden severe distortion of the visual image from the affected eye. There is no pain. Flashes of light or the perception of dark moving or floating objects may be seen. As further separation occurs there may be the perception of a curtain or veil followed by severe distortion of the images. Retinal detachment occurs almost exclusively in a single eye, so the image in the opposite eye remains normal.

That is a severe medical emergency requiring the care of a retinologist, if one is available. Hospitalization is usually required. Tears in the retina can be repaired, usually by means of laser surgery. The detached retina is usually forced back into its normal position by means of a bubble of gas that is introduced into the bulb of the eye, increasing the pressure within the eye. In most cases there is a good chance for recovery of vision.

MACULAR DEGENERATION

Incidence and Distribution

This condition has been seen with increasing frequency in the twenty first century. It occurs chiefly in people over the age of fifty and is now the greatest single cause of blindness in people over sixty five in the U.S. That is due in part to the fact that people are living longer for various reasons that have been given earlier. Macular degeneration occurs in both sexes, somewhat more in men than in women, although the predisposition for the disease is passed in the female chromosome. The cause of macular degeneration is not known. There is definitely a congenital aspect, as macular degeneration is frequently seen in families.

Pathophysiology of Macular Degeneration

It is of extreme curiosity that the part of the retina that is involved is the macula, that very central point where there is the greatest concentration of cones. The periphery of the retina, containing mainly the rods is unaffected. The result is that one loses the ability to read and to see small images. That includes newsprint, and other small close images and larger images seen from a greater distance, such as street signs. That is the chief reason why this disease is the main cause of loss of the ability to safely drive an automobile.

There are two types of macular degeneration: wet and dry. In the "wet" type there is active bleeding in the vascular layer of the retina. In some cases that is related to "drusen", fatty globules, on the vascular bed, causing vessels to rupture. The term "Dry" macular degeneration describes a state of atrophy of the cones, probably as the result of earlier bleeding. In either form there is loss of vision. The extent of visual loss depends on the extent of damage to the cones.

This disease usually begins in a single eye, but in most cases extends to the opposite eye also. It is not uncommon to have the loss of vision much more severe in one eye than in the other.

Treatment of Macular Degeneration

The treatment of macular degeneration is in a state of evolution at this time. Many research protocols have been tried, most with little success. Many projects are under way at this time. There has been some success in treatment of the wet type by the use of a combination of a chemical compound and low-level laser radiation. It is referred to as "Photodynamic Therapy." A photosensitive compound is injected into an arm vein, and then travels to all parts of the body, including the affected retina. With the use of an ophthalmic telescope the operator sees the injected material enter the blood vessels of the involved macular area, and then radiates the area with a low energy laser. The laser radiation activates the material, which then seals off the bleeding capillaries, stopping the bleeding. That treatment has been successful, but in many cases needs to be repeated periodically.

There is no successful treatment for dry macular degeneration at this time. Many approaches have been tried with little success. At the time of this writing there is a promising treatment involving the injection of medication into the bulb of the eye. This study, using a product called Lucentis, showed the ability to stop bleeding in a "wet" eye. Early results suggest that, if treated early enough in the course of the disease, "dry macular degeneration" might be prevented, thus greatly improving the prospects for avoiding blindness.

Macular degeneration is certainly the most serious and threatening eye disease for the senior population today.

DIABETIC RETINOPATHY

This disease is the chief cause of blindness in people under the age of sixty in the United States. Diabetics who are in poor control are the most likely to become totally blind. Some degree of loss of vision is not uncommon in most diabetics. Diabetes in children which manifests itself earlier in life tends to be a more aggressive form of diabetes than the adult, or late onset form of diabetes. In the earlier chapter on diabetes mellitus it was stated that the worst systemic effects of that disease are caused mainly by the damage done to the very small blood vessels throughout the body. The process of atherosclerosis accelerated and magnified by diabetes causes the capillaries and arterioles to become blocked. In the eyes the main target of diabetes is the vascular layer of the retina. Arterioles become blocked with the fatty material of atherosclerosis and fail to conduct blood to the cones and rods. Those structures that are deprived of their blood supply die. The result is the loss of vision from the area of the retina supplied by the diseased vessel. That loss is permanent.

Treatment of diabetic retinopathy must be directed mainly at the prevention and control of diabetes. That requires a vigorous program of education to get people to eat less and exercise more. There is absolutely no doubt of the connection between obesity and diabetes, especially in juveniles and people of African descent.

In the case of arterial bleeding and venous thrombosis within the eye due to diabetic retinopathy intervention by a retinologist can be very helpful.

GLAUCOMA

Glaucoma is the second most common cause of blindness in the United States. The disease is manifested by increase in pressure within the eye, (intra-ocular pressure). It most often occurs in one eye at a time, although both eyes are ultimately involved in most cases. The true underlying cause of glaucoma is not known. Predisposing factors include age over sixty, although it is also seen in much younger people, in people with hypertension, extreme myopia, and people of African descent.

In the normal eye a clear fluid called aqueous humor is produced by a structure called the ciliary body of the eye. That fluid is circulated throughout the chambers of the eye, carrying oxygen, nutrients, and waste products to and from all structures of the eye. The production of aqueous humor is continuous, as is the excretion of waste aqueous humor. The route of excretion is through the anterior chamber of the eye, into specialized channels.

The cause of the increase in intra-ocular pressure is a disturbance in the outflow of aqueous humor. Overproduction is theoretically one of the causes of glaucoma. The anterior chamber of the normal eye has openings through which the aqueous humor leaves the eye. In glaucoma those openings become narrowed, restricting the outflow, although the production continues at a normal rate. The resulting increase in volume creates an increase in pressure within the eye.

That pressure, if not corrected can severely damage the optic nerve, resulting in partial or complete blindness. There are two types of glaucoma, referred to as open angle, or closed angle glaucoma, depending upon the abnormality in the anterior chamber.

The symptoms and signs of glaucoma usually include some awareness of clouding, or loss of vision which becomes progressively more severe if ignored. In some cases there is redness or pain and tenderness of the eye. A visit to an ophthalmologist can reveal the presence of increased intra-ocular pressure. Treatment can be instituted. Topical medication in the form of eye drops is usually very effective, and is continued thereafter. In some cases surgical treatment is required. Modern surgical treatment in most cases is done with laser, and has a good rate of success.

RETINITIS PIGMENTOSA

This is a disease of congenital origin. The exact mechanism of genetic transmission is not certain. It does not usually involve multiple members of a family. There is no known metabolic or infectious cause.

The disease involves both eyes. It usually manifests itself early in life and becomes progressively more severe, causing blindness in most cases. The underlying process is the deposition of black melanin pigment in the visual layer of the retina. The rod cells are the first to become involved, resulting in loss of peripheral vision and night and low-light vision. As the disease progresses the cones become involved, with the loss of central fine discrimination vision. As the deposition of pigment continues the loss of vision becomes complete. At this time there is no known cure for retinitis pigmentosa. The end-result is usually total blindness.

THE EARS—ORGANS OF HEARING AND EQUILIBRIUM

The ears and related structures serve two distinct and very important functions. They are the organs of hearing and the organs of balance and equilibrium. There are three anatomical divisions; the external ear, the middle ear and the inner ear. The hearing apparatus is in the external, middle and a portion of the inner ear. The apparatus of equilibrium is entirely within the inner ear.

The External Ear

The external ear is covered with skin overlying a framework of cartilage with the exception of the soft ear lobes. The cartilage framework is exquisitely shaped to capture sound waves and to direct them into the ear canal which is lined with skin. At the inner end of the ear canal is the tympanic membrane, commonly called the eardrum. That name is very appropriate because the tympanic membrane is a sheet of tissue that is modified skin. It is tightly adherent to every contour of the ear canal, making an airtight seal. The physical impact of sound waves coming through the ear canal causes the tympanic membrane to vibrate in the same way as a drumhead when struck. The speed and amplitude of the vibrations vary with those of the sound waves entering the ear.

The Middle Ear

The middle ear lies within the temporal bone of the skull. It is a closed chamber that is filled with air that comes from the inner opening of the Eustachean tube. The outer wall of the middle ear is the tympanic membrane. The inner wall is the foramen ovale, or oval window, that constitutes the outer wall of the inner ear.

Extending through the middle ear chamber are three tiny bones, named from antiquity the incus, (anvil), malleus, (hammer), and stapes, (stirrup), because of their physical appearance and their functions. Those bones are actually connected by joints. The malleus is connected to the tympanic membrane, the stapes to the foramen ovale, and the incus connects the two. The vibrations of the tympanic membrane are transmitted by the malleus to the incus which transmits them to the stapes. The vibrations are transmitted by the stapes to the foramen ovale, and through that opening into the inner ear.

The middle ear is a closed chamber except for a small opening in its medial wall which is the entrance to the Eustachean tube. That is the name given, also in antiquity, to a canal that extends through the temporal bone of the skull, opening at its medial end into the nasopharynx. The Eustachean tube is the only means of equalizing the pressure within the middle ear. That becomes very important if we experience changes in barometric pressure, as in SCUBA diving, or ascending in a non-pressurized aircraft. The inner opening of the Eustachean tube can become blocked by swelling of the mucous membrane of the nasopharynx due to allergy or infection or enlargement of the tonsils. That can lead to serious problems, as we will see later in this chapter.

The Inner Ear

The oval window separates the middle ear from the inner ear. Both structures lie within the protection of the temporal bone of the skull. The oval window is actually the end piece of a structure called the cochlea, so named in Greek because that is the word for the shell of a snail, which the cochlea resembles. It is a coiled tube, filled with fluid called the endolymph. The widest portion of the cochlea is at the oval window and it gradually narrows to its point of termination.

The movement of the three bones within the middle ear is converted by the vibration of the oval window to fluid waves within the endolymph of the cochlea. The cochlea is lined with a basement membrane containing many very small nerves. Extending from the basement membrane into the lumen of the cochlea is a series of tiny hair-like projections, called hair cells. The hair cells are the longest at the widest end of the cochlea near the oval window, and become progressively shorter as the diameter of the cochlea diminishes. Each hair cell is rooted in the basement membrane and ultimately makes connection with a single tiny nerve in the basement membrane.

The hair cells are flexible and vibrate in response to the physical energy of the fluid waves within the cochlea. The longest hair cells respond to the lowest pitched sound waves and the shortest hair cells to the highest pitched sound waves. The vibration of the hair cells stimulates the structures of the basement membrane at their roots. The physical energy of the vibrating hair cell causes a chemical reaction to occur. The compound ATP is reduced to one called ADP in the same reaction as that which occurs in the retina of the eye. This reaction causes the release of a tiny amount of electrical energy. That energy is picked up by the nerve at the base of the hair cell and communicated to progressively larger nerves, ultimately to a large nerve called the acoustic nerve which goes directly to the hearing center of the brain. The simultaneous nerve input of thousands of hair cells from each ear is relayed to the centers of the brain that decode the messages and scrutinize them through the memory center for recognition. That information is then relayed to the center of the cerebral cortex that decides what to do with the information.

Thus the hearing process requires conversion from physical energy to chemical energy to electrical energy to nerve impulses. All of this is done in milliseconds on an unconscious level.

The organ of balance and equilibrium is adjacent to the cochlea. It consists of three gracefully looping tubular structures, set at angles precisely suited to encompass all positions of the head. They are called the semicircular canals. Within each canal is a basement membrane containing nerves and blood vessels. Projecting into the lumen of each semicircular canal are hair-like projections called cilia which have their bases in the nerve cells of the basement membrane. The semicircular canals are filled with a fluid called otolymph. Suspended in the otolymph are multiple small solid particles called otoliths. The otoliths are free to roll and move about within the semicircular canals as the position of the head changes. Their movements are transmitted to the nerve cells in the basement membrane by the rolling and bumping of the otoliths into the cilia.

At that point a process takes place that is similar to that within the cochlea. The movement of the otoliths stimulates the nerves within the basement membrane, causing the breakdown of ATP to ADP, with the release of a minute amount of electrical energy. That energy stimulates the nerves within the basement membrane. Those nerve fibers terminate in a nerve that relays information about position of the head and body to the cerebellar brain center that then processes the information. If the nerve input becomes excessive one becomes aware of the sensation of motion sickness.

The foregoing was a simplistic description of the function of a tiny organ that is immensely important to the function of the body. The information relayed to the brain gives a moment- to- moment accounting of the position of the body. It is closely integrated with information from the eyes that is simultaneously relayed from the optic nerves to the brain. That combined information acts as a gyroscopic control of the position of the head and body. It is integrated instantaneously to enable a gymnast or acrobat to perform precise movements and to hold positions. It is essential to all of us to stabilize our movements and to be aware of our position in relation to our environment.

A very common example or the importance of this mechanism is that of being in a moving vehicle, such as a boat or in a car on a twisty road. The constant change of position of the head causes excessive movements of the otoliths within the semicircular canals. That information, relayed to the brain, causes the malady that we know as motion sickness. The result is a sense of severe unease, dizziness, and nausea, which often leads to vomiting. The reasons for the latter are not clear, but are open to speculation, such as a form of the alarm reaction, activating the autonomic nervous system to prepare the body to deal with that emergency by emptying the stomach, however inappropriate it appears.

An example of how the brain enables us to compensate for unfavorable states such as being car sick or seasick is that of a passenger in a car or boat who experiences motion sickness. If that passenger is given the wheel or the helm and is required to follow the movements of the vehicle with his or her eyes the state of disequilibrium often passes. Of course this is not possible if one is a passenger in a ship or a bus, or is required to remain in the rear seat of a car.

COMMON DISORDERS OF THE EAR

Disorders of the External Ear

"Never put anything smaller than your elbow in your ear!" (Kindergarten Advice)

The external ear is composed chiefly of cartilage and skin. With the exception of birth defects and injuries not much can go wrong with the cartilage framework of the outer ear. The skin, however, can have many of the problems that affect the skin anywhere in the body, including rash eruptions, infections and cancer. The external ear canal is lined with very soft and fragile skin containing an abundance of oil producing glands. There does not seem to be any good reason for that, other than to lubricate that skin. However the oil glands in many people produce an over-abundance of thick oil that dries and thickens to form ear wax, properly called cerumen. In many people the wax accumulates to the point where it obstructs the ear canal, resulting in partial or complete loss of hearing. When that occurs it is necessary to remove the thick wax.

Here is where the most common of ear problems is encountered. Because the skin lining the external ear canal never sees the light of day it is very soft and has no protection against friction and other injuries of most skin areas. Efforts to clean wax out of the ears result in a multitude of visits to the doctor for ear infections. This is where the common sense advice given to most kindergarten children is useful: "never put anything smaller than your elbow into your ear." Wax can usually be irrigated out with warm water, using a soft rubber bulb syringe. A trained person should treat more resistant cases.

Another skin problem of the external ear is the formation of cysts that contain dehydrated and concentrated skin oil. They are called "sebaceous cysts." Those cysts can become infected and be very painful, but are easily treated in the hands of experienced personnel.

There is one disorder of the external auditory canal that is unique to surfers and others who swim in cold water. For reasons that are not clear they develop bony prominences in the subcutaneous bone of the external ear canal. Those prominences, sometimes casually referred to as "surfers' ears" narrow the width of the canal, causing obstruction of the drainage of oil and wax from the ear, often leading to obstruction with wax. Surgical removal of the bony projections is sometimes necessary.

The eardrum rarely has problems of its own other than accidental injuries and perforations. It can be very severely involved in problems that occur in the middle ear, which will be discussed next. That leaves only one frequently seen problem involving the external ear:

foreign bodies inserted into the ear canal, usually by small children. The most common first signs and symptoms are fever and earache with loss of hearing which occurs at some time after the insertion of the foreign object. It can be a very severe and serious problem, requiring the services of an ear specialist to remove the foreign object.

Disorders of the Middle Ear

The most common problem is infection which is referred to as Otitis Media. This occurs most often as the result of a respiratory infection involving the nose and throat. In our anatomical tour we saw that the Eustachean tube is the only passageway in or out of the closed box of the middle ear. That tube travels through the mastoid bone with one opening in the middle ear and the other in the nasopharynx. Quite frequently the mucous membrane of the nasopharynx becomes extremely swollen because of local infection. That swelling can quite easily cause complete obstruction of the inner opening of the Eustachean tube. When that happens two things can occur. First is the loss of ability of the middle ear to adjust to changes in barometric pressure. That causes earache and dullness of hearing. Secondly, the infecting organism that caused swelling of the mucous membrane of the nasopharynx can enter the Eustachian tube and can travel into the middle ear, causing an infection of that chamber. That infection is referred to as otitis media. The usual signs and symptoms are earache, fever and loss of hearing in that ear. Otitis media occasionally involves both ears but usually involves only one ear at a time.

Otitis media is a serious problem, usually requiring medical attention. The eardrum is frequently involved, becoming red and bulging outward or inwardly retracted, depending on the pressure changes in the middle ear. The eardrum may rupture spontaneously if the pressure within the middle ear becomes too great. In many cases it is necessary to make an opening in the eardrum in order to reduce the pressure within the middle ear and permit drainage. In chronic cases of closure of the Eustachean tube it is often necessary to insert a small tube through an opening in the ear drum for prolonged periods until the internal swelling of the nasopharyngeal end of the Eustachean tube subsides.

In cases of severe otitis media with prolonged inflammation there may be an accumulation of serum or blood within the middle ear. That is referred to as an effusion. Because of the sticky nature of serum and of blood cells this may act as glue, enveloping the bones of the middle ear. The final result of such an effusion may be that the bones fail to function normally, causing hearing loss. To correct that condition requires a surgical procedure to free the bones. There is usually a good result from such surgery, but in some cases there may be permanent impairment of hearing. Another serious condition involving the middle ear is otosclerosis, which actually is an arthritic process involving the tiny joints connecting two or more of the three bones. This condition is not rare and usually can be significantly improved with surgery.

The type of deafness that results from the above disorders of the eardrum and the middle ear is referred to as "conduction deafness", because of the loss of ability of the ear to conduct sound waves into the inner ear, which is the ultimate hearing organ. We will next discuss some of the disorders that affect the inner ear.

Disorders of the Inner Ear

Failure of any hearing component of the inner ear causes the hearing loss called "nerve deafness." It is the most common form of hearing loss because it most often occurs in people past middle age at which time we are all subject to the changes of the aging process. The chief among those is atherosclerosis.

The arteries of the basement membrane of the cochlea are extremely small, yet are subject to the same atherosclerotic process as any of the larger arteries in the body. They can become progressively more obstructed to the point at which they are completely blocked. The result is the loss of blood supply and the death of the hair cells and nerves at their bases. Another frequent cause of permanent "nerve deafness" is the chronic exposure to loud noises, such as jet engine noise or working in a noisy metal factory without wearing ear protective gear.

Nerve deafness is treated chiefly with one or another types of hearing aids. The science of audiology has improved greatly in recent years since the advent of the understanding of digital sound reproduction. Modern hearing aids are available in many basic designs, some pre-programmed and others equipped with controls allowing the user to make many adjustments. Most people with nerve deafness can benefit from properly prescribed hearing aids. There are other causes of hearing loss due to failure of an inner ear component, but they are not commonly seen.

Tinnitus

That is the name given to a disorder in which one perceives a sound that is generated by a defect within the hearing organ. The sound is usually a high-pitched whistle or hissing noise, but can also be a lower-pitched note. It is continuous when one "tunes in" on it, but frequently is not heard when one's attention is diverted away from the sound. That is the case in most people with tinnitus. Tinnitus usually occurs in one ear initially, but most often progresses to involve both ears. There is usually some hearing loss when the disorder becomes chronic.

Tinnitus can occur following exposure to a very loud noise, such as an electronic pop or squeal while wearing headphones, or the sound of a gun, or an explosion. However, in most cases there is usually no such trauma involved, but rather the same cause as was stated for nerve deafness in the previous section. That is the loss of blood supply to a section of the cochlear hairs due to atherosclerosis. As the blood supply diminishes that part of the hearing organ becomes irritated, initiating the false perception of sound. In the latter case the sound of tinnitus has been poetically described as "the death scream of dying neurons."

In most cases tinnitus lasts for the person's lifetime. Many forms of treatment have been offered. Some are partially successful in reducing the intensity of the sound for a while, but there is no known cure that is practical. In the great majority of cases the person afflicted learns to live with the disorder. There are very rare instances in which the sound of tinnitus is truly intolerable. In those cases the only recourse is to destroy the hearing organ of the ear most seriously affected, causing deafness in that ear. That treatment, to be sure, is very rarely used.

Disequilibrium

This name is used to describe the condition in which one's sense of balance and perception of spatial relationships is disturbed or defective. It is most commonly due to an affliction of the semicircular canal balance center in one ear. In rare cases the cause is a stroke or other disorder involving the cerebellum of the brain that perceives balance and equilibrium. There is recent interest in the possibility that disequilibrium can be a manifestation of an auto-immune disorder affecting the balance center of the ear or the brain itself. That study has not yet been completed.

Disequilibrium is so commonly experienced that there are a number of medications available, both by prescription and over the counter to relieve that condition. Most of those are effective in all but the most severe cases. A favorite prescription medication is the transdermal scopolamine patch. A warning should always be stated that scopolamine is a very powerful medication that can cause severe agitation and disorientation in susceptible individuals. In most cases over- the- counter Dramamine or Bonamine are effective and quite safe, other than causing drowsiness.

It is very important to note that if disequilibrium suddenly appears in an individual who is not actually in a state of rapidly moving or being tossed about in a boat it may be due to a problem at the other end of the line; the brain. A stroke involving the cerebellar region can produce all of the above changes, either alone, or accompanied by loss of consciousness or other major signs and symptoms. The sudden appearance of those symptoms must be reported to your physician as soon as possible. It may be worth going to an E.R. for immediate investigation.

Meniere's Disease

The name was given in 1868 in honor of the French physician who first described this disorder. It is a state of disequilibrium that appears suddenly with no apparent cause, usually accompanied by tinnitus and some hearing loss. It is most often seen in people over the age of fifty, but can occur at an earlier age. It is usually unilateral, but with the passage of time can become bilateral. It can last for a year or a lifetime. The cause is unknown, but recent research has shown some relationship to auto-immune disease.

Meniere's disease is usually manifested by acute attacks of severe loss of equilibrium in which the individual loses balance and may fall to the floor, out of control. The attacks may last from moments to hours. They are usually accompanied by one-sided tinnitus. The attacks may be only occasional or very frequent. Tinnitus and hearing loss are associated with persistence of the above symptoms over some length of time.

There is no known method of prevention of the attacks. Suppression of the labyrinth of the inner ear with oral or transdermal medications may help in mild cases. Severe cases may require some type of surgical procedure. Ongoing care by a medical specialist trained in this type of disorder is usually required.

THE SENSES OF TOUCH AND PAIN

Touch

The sense organ of touch is located in the skin on every surface of the body. The nerve endings for touch are in the dermis layer of the skin which is the layer just deep to the surface layer, the epidermis. The skin throughout the body is supplied with these nerve endings. They are "on duty" every minute of the day and night, perceiving every touch and relaying the messages to the brain. Fortunately, the brain has the capacity to be aware of those millions of messages that come in to it continuously and to screen out the vast majority of those messages, monitoring the normal input of the external contacts with the skin. Any new and different input catches the brain's attention and is immediately examined.

In order for an input of touch to be forwarded to the brain's level of awareness it must be either a different message from those that are received normally, or the response to a prior command from the brain to feel something.

There are areas of the skin in which there is a greater concentration of sensory nerve endings than in other areas of the body. One example is those areas that have been labeled "the erogenous zones." They include the genitals, the nipples and the lips in most people. Any individual may have his or her personal erogenous zones based on personal variations in anatomical development, or preference due to past experience.

Probably the most impressive example of increased touch sensitivity is in the fingertips. In most individuals the ability to perceive touch can be improved through training. A perfect example is the ability to read Braille printing by people who have lost the sense of sight. Braille printing is in the form of series of raised dots on a page. By learning to scan those dots with fingertips people can become able to read rapidly with good comprehension.

What Can Go Wrong With the Sense of Touch?

A severe burn or deep abrasion can destroy the sensory nerve endings in the affected area of skin. In most cases this results in a temporary loss or distortion of touch until the area heals completely. With complete healing the sense of touch is usually restored. In the case of very extensive and deep local injuries that destroy the dermis layer completely touch can be lost permanently in the affected area.

Laceration wounds that sever sensory nerves in any area can result in the loss of all sensation from the point of injury distally to the area of skin served by that sensory nerve. . In the case of small nerve trunks in the fingers or toes this can result in complete loss of touch sensation for a long period of time, but such sensory nerves usually heal within their myelin sheathes and sensation is finally restored. In the case of major injury to large sensory nerve trunks in any extremity the loss of sensation to the entire extremity distal to the laceration can result, and can be permanent unless surgical repair is done.

Injury to the brain, such as trauma, stroke or tumor affecting the area where sensory messages are received can result in extensive and permanent loss of sensation to the area from which the messages originated. Finally, demyelinating diseases such as multiple sclerosis can cause patchy loss of sensation in multiple areas of the body. That kind of loss is also permanent

Pain

The sense of pain is different from the sense of touch in that it involves areas of the brain that are not usually involved in touch perception and different nerve pathways with receptor nerves that are specific for pain. Pain perception is often but not exclusively carried by the pathways of touch. One example of that is the situation in which one's finger touches something very hot. The local touch receptor nerves sense the heat, and then adjacent nerves join in that sensation. That is called "recruitment of nerves." The message is sent to the brain as more than simple touch sensation. That message is immediately relayed to the pain center of the brain. The memory and association centers come into play and the message is sent to the motor center as a call for action. The motor center then orders the appropriate muscles to contract, pulling the finger away from the hot object.

Another and completely different scenario is that of deep pain. If an injurious event occurs, such as a sprain, or fracture or the passage of a kidney stone there are local pain receptor nerves that are stimulated. Those nerves send a message directly to the pain center of the brain.

That message is then relayed to the memory and association centers. At this point we encounter another concept of pain.

There are two major kinds of pain: acute and chronic pain. The pain described above, in which the finger touches a hot object, or the pain of a kidney stone, is acute pain. The response of pulling the finger away from danger is an appropriate acute or immediate response.

An example of chronic pain is that in which the cause of the pain has been present for some time. Examples would be a cancer that causes pain, or the pain due to a herniated disc in the low back. In those conditions the local pain receptor nerves send more or less continuous pain messages to the brain. The pain center of the brain relays the messages to the memory and association centers which recognize the pain as being "old news", or chronic pain. The higher association center makes the decision that no motor action would be appropriate, and no motor response follows. Severe chronic pain usually requires some type of remedy, either surgical or medical.

It is the author's opinion that the sense of pain should be listed as a sixth sense, in addition to the five senses listed at the beginning of this chapter. The distinction between acute pain and chronic pain illustrates how complex some sensations are that are carried through the neural pathways that serve the sense of touch in normal conditions. Different receptors in the brain and different emotional reactions are involved in the two kinds of pain.

The individual's ability or inability to accommodate to chronic pain is quite different from the usual reaction to acute pain. The medical specialty of Pain Management is a fairly recent addition to the disciplines of medicine and is very important in the day-to-day lives of people who live in chronic pain.

THE SENSE OF SMELL

The receptor organ for the sense of smell consists of clumps of highly specialized tissue located high in the septal side of the nasal passages. As in the case of the senses of sight and hearing the receptors are small structures consisting of a chemical side and a neural or electrical side. Incoming airborne particles come in contact with these tissues and initiate a complicated series of events. The aerosols are in a sense digested, initiating a complex chemical reaction, as in the senses of sight and hearing. Chemical compounds are broken down, releasing small amounts of energy from the receptor organ. That energy is transformed from chemical energy into electrical energy in the form of electrons. That energy is perceived by a specialized receptor and fed into synaptic nerve endings. Those nerve fibers ultimately lead to a large nerve called the olfactory nerve. That nerve goes to the olfactory center of the brain.

From the olfactory receiving center of the brain the messages in the form of nerve impulses are relayed to the memory center for recognition, then to the association area for response. The messages can be pleasant, as in the form of food smells or scents from other sources, or unpleasant, as in the case of noxious odors.

It is in the memory and association areas of the brain that the education process occurs. By repeated exposures we learn to recognize smells and to assign to them good or bad connotations. The result can be avoidance of "bad" smells or pleasure in identifying and enjoying the "good" smells. All of this, as in the other senses, occurs within milliseconds of perceiving the smells.

A very high degree of education of the ability to smell is possible, as in the example of perfume testers or others whose occupations consist of identifying and selecting or improving products based on their scents.

What Can Go Wrong With the Sense of Smell?

Anosmia, which is the proper scientific name for loss of the sense of smell, can be due to multiple causes. The first is a congenital defect in which one is born without the sense of smell. That can be due to either an abnormality of the receptors in the nose or to a problem with the nerve pathway to the brain, or to a defect in the brain itself. That is a very rare condition for which there is no explanation and no cure. Severe chronic infections of the nose or other chronic inflammatory diseases that affect the mucous membrane bearing the organs of smell can cause anosmia.

A far more common cause is the chronic use of topical nasal decongestants. Those preparations, used in moderation for only a few days are helpful in relieving nasal congestion. However, some are powerful vasoconstrictors that cause reduction of the blood supply to the mucous membrane. With prolonged use the nasal mucosa becomes severely inflamed, leading to the formation of scar tissue and damage to the organs of smell.

By far the worst damage to the organs of smell is inflicted by the chronic nasal inhalation of cocaine or similar narcotic substances. The result of that habit is severe chronic inflammation and scarring of the mucous membrane and the loss of the sense of smell, in many cases the loss is permanent.

It is very unfortunate that at the present state of the art there is no effective remedy for anosmia due to any of the above causes. It is very true that our enjoyment of the taste of food is closely linked with the enjoyment of the smell of the food. That cannot be replaced. Also, the benefit of being warned against spoiled food by its smell and the ability to avoid noxious substances by their smell cannot be restored.

Another reason for loss of the sense of smell is some damage to the brain involving the olfactory center, or the memory center, or also the centers of association and cognition. All of those parts of the brain are necessary for the maintenance of an effective sense of smell. A tumor or stroke in those areas can cause loss of the ability to smell.

Another phenomenon also occurs in some cases. Some seizure disorders, the spontaneous firing off of neurons in the olfactory area of the brain can cause the patient to have the sensation of smelling an odor that is not really there, but is generated by the stimulation of nerve pathways due to the seizure. If in the course of a seizure the patient experiences a strong smell, usually described as a bad or offensive smell a strong clue is delivered as to the probable location of the of the irritant causing the seizure.

THE SENSE OF TASTE

Scientists tell us that there are five "primary taste sensations." They are: salty, sweet, sour, bitter, and umami. The first four are familiar to us all. The fifth taste, umami, refers to the response to the salts of glutamic acid. An easy instance of that is MSG (monosodium glutamate), a flavor enhancer frequently added to prepared foods and a favorite of Chinese restaurants.

The receptors for the sense of taste are the taste buds. Those small organs are located on the tongue and the adjacent walls of the pharynx. They function in much the same way as the receptors for the sense of smell.

Substances that enter the mouth come in contact with the taste buds. They are, in a sense, digested by the taste buds. Chemical reactions occur in which the substances are broken down to their chemical constituents. Those compounds are then analyzed by the receptors in the taste buds. Chemical reactions occur in which there is the breakdown of compounds with the resultant release of electrons. Those electrons stimulate microscopic synaptic nerve endings in the taste buds. Those nerve stimuli are gathered into a nerve bundle that travels to the brain.

Within the brain the messages from the taste buds are first received in the center for taste reception. From there they are forwarded to the memory center for recognition, then to the association center for the discrimination of the kind of tastes they are. Decisions are made as to the "good", or "bad" quality of the tastes, and then to the higher centers of the cerebrum for further directions as to whether to eat and enjoy the substances, or to reject them.

As in the case of the sense of smell, it should be remembered that all of these processes take place within milliseconds from the time the food substances enter the mouth. It should also be kept in mind that with very few exceptions, tastes and smells are subject to screening by the association center of the brain, and there judged by the memory of previous exposures and experiences to be either favorable or unfavorable. It has been said that chocolate is one of the few substances that is universally liked and craved. It certainly gets the vote of this author.

The mechanism of the sense of taste is essentially the same in people of all cultures. The enjoyment, appreciation, and craving for certain foods or beverages are the result of learning. There are cultural tastes, based upon the way one was raised, and there are individual tastes, based upon one's experience. The food tastes of China are far different from those of Mexico, or Norway. Yet, the taste apparatus is the same for people of all of those cultures. They are all the result of a learning experience.

Excellent examples of the power of education of taste are the professional wine and food tasters who can identify the food or wine they are tasting, and give the ingredients, the origin, and in the case of wine, the nationality, region, and even the precise location of the vineyard. It should be noted that there is a significant variation in the number and quality of taste buds that are genetically conferred. There are "hyper-tasters" who have significantly more taste buds than most people, and therefore have a greater ability to define, remember, and describe various tastes. The same applies to individuals who are "hyper-smellers." Those individuals frequently find employment in industries in which their abilities are valued.

What Can Go Wrong With the Sense Of Taste?

As in the case of the sense of smell, one can be born without the sense of taste, due to a congenital abnormality of some sort. Fortunately, that is very rare and is an incurable condition.

Any severe intra-oral burn, whether thermal or chemical can very severely injure the taste buds and cause a loss of the sense of taste. Fortunately, in most cases the affected structures on the tongue and walls of the pharynx usually heal and the sense of taste is restored.

Disorders of the brain can cause loss of the sense of taste. That loss is usually permanent. Such cases are very rare. As was mentioned earlier, severe loss of the sense of smell can greatly affect the sense of taste.

Chapter Nine
THE SKIN

OVERVIEW

The entire skin of the body, including hair and nails, is classed and treated as a single organ consisting of various parts. It is the largest organ of the body in terms of area and it serves a variety of essential functions. They include:

1. A COVERING FOR THE BODY
2. A SENSORY ORGAN (touch)
3. A REGULATOR OF BODY TEMPERATURE (sweat and insulation)
4. A PROTECTOR AGAINST INJURY (callus formation, hands and feet, finger nails and toenails)
5. AN ORGAN OF NUTRITION (making vitamin D upon exposure to sunlight)
6. AN ORGAN OF BEAUTY (universal in all cultures)
7. A SCENT GLAND (the apocrine glands)

All of the functions of the skin listed above are, in general, self-explanatory and need no further elaboration with the exception of the skin as an organ of scent. That function is due to very highly specialized sweat glands that are located in the axillae, (armpits) and the perianal region (immediately surrounding the anus). Those are named "the apocrine glands." The ordinary sweat glands that are distributed throughout most of the skin secrete sweat in response to exercise and in hot weather as a means of cooling the body by the evaporation of the sweat.

Apocrine glands are much larger than sweat glands elsewhere in the body. They have a very rich supply of nerve endings that originate in the autonomic nervous system. They secrete a copious thick fluid that has a strong acrid odor at times of high emotional states. They have no function in cooling the body. One can be in a very cold room but if under a high level of emotional stress the apocrine glands can pour forth a copious secretion that is very different from the odor of sweat from other areas of the skin.

These specialized glands are seen in some other mammals in which they serve as a means of communicating sexual excitement, or fear, or simply anxiety. Others recognize the scent as a non-verbal communication of those emotional states. That form of communication occurs in humans and is important in some cultures.

THE ANATOMY OF THE SKIN

The skin is essentially composed of two layers: the epidermis, which is the outermost layer, and the dermis, located immediately deep to the epidermis. The two layers are very different from each other microscopically and have very different functions.

The epidermis is actually composed of five layers of cells. The deepest layer contains basal cells from which all the other cells mature in layers. The most superficial layer is composed of flattened cells containing much keratin, a hard protein. That surface layer serves as a protective layer. Its plate-like cells are in various stages of maturation and dying and are shed continuously.

Every time we bathe and towel off we remove a huge number of dead surface cells. In people who habitually do hard manual work, or walk barefoot the hands and feet can be covered with callus. That name is given to thickened surface corium cells set in a base of keratin. Callus confers a rough, horny layer of protection to those areas.

Most people, especially ladies, strive to keep their hands and other epidermal areas soft by means of lotions and scrubs which are included in the vast industry of skin care preparations.

Fingernails and hair are composed chiefly of keratin supporting an infrastructure of plate-like epithelial cells. They represent a very highly specialized form of epidermal epithelium that grows continuously. The color of hair and skin is conferred by black melanin pigment that is also manufactured in the basal portion of the epidermal layer. The density of the melanin pigment gives skin and hair its color. The same melanin pigment is present in the iris of the eye and is responsible for the color of the eyes. Racial genetics determine the density of pigment and therefore the color of skin and hair in various individuals. Exposure to sunlight increases the color density of melanin in the skin. That is called the tanning effect.

At the base of the epidermal layer is the basement membrane. That membrane gives rise to the epithelial cells of the epidermis, and also to the melanin pigment. The basement membrane separates the epidermis from the dermis.

The dermis layer is thicker than the epidermis and is much more complex. Within the dermis lie the nerves that give us the sense of touch. Also in that layer are the blood vessels that provide nutrition and remove the waste products of metabolism from the skin. The sweat glands are also housed in the dermis and also the apocrine scent glands. The hair follicles are in the dermal layer, giving rise to the hair shafts that penetrate the epidermal layer through small tunnels. The sebaceous glands that produce the oil that lubricates the skin are also within the dermis. Their oil is conducted to the surface of the epidermis through small conduits of their own.

Lying just below the basement layer of the dermis is the fat layer of the body. Subcutaneous fat encases the entire body. It is an essential part of our anatomy. It is supplied with blood vessels and metabolizes just as do all the other parts of the body.

Along with the deep stores of fat that are present within the abdominal cavity subcutaneous fat is our storage site of unused calories of energy. That is a graphic demonstration of the first law of thermodynamics: energy cannot be created or destroyed but is transformed into a different form of energy. Fat is a form of protection against starvation in times of famine, or in conditions of great privation. It also works the other way: if the caloric intake exceeds the amount of calories consumed in the functions of the body the excess of calories are converted to fat, which is stored away.

In some, but not all people the subcutaneous layer of fat becomes reduced with the passage of the years. That causes thinning of the face and neck and of the extremities. The result is a change in physical appearance, with wrinkling of the skin and the appearance of skin folds and lines. When that happens the skin becomes more fragile, bruising more easily and is more susceptible to scrapes and tears. Those are unavoidable and unpreventable attributes of aging in some people.

COMMON DISORDERS OF THE SKIN

Dermatitis

Dermatitis is the name given to rashes and eruptions of the skin. That term applies to infections and inflammation of the skin due to a number of varied causes. We will discuss them according to the causes of each.

Contact Dermatitis

Contact dermatitis is among the most common types of skin eruption. It is caused by contact with specific irritants. In most cases the location of the eruption on specific body parts and the description of the eruptions provide strong clues to the diagnosis. For example: one's hands come in contact with irritating detergents or solvents and there is a rash, localized to the area of contact. The exposed skin is usually reddened and there may be a puffy patchy swelling of the area which commonly called "hives." The medical term for hives is "urticaria." The eruption will be itchy. The location and description of the eruption tells us to look for a causative agent that came in contact with that specific area of skin.

Another type of contact dermatitis is that from allergenic contact. This is typified by touching plants that secrete a highly irritating and allergenic substance, such as poison oak or poison ivy. There the rash may be patchy, involving each part of the skin that made contact with the leaves. The rash can be similar to that described above with redness and urticaria, and may also appear as blisters containing blood serum. In the case of poison ivy or oak there may be some of the allergenic substance remaining on one's clothing or shoes. If that substance comes in contact with the skin it will cause a new focus of skin eruption. A very easily diagnosed cause of contact dermatitis is nickel. Some people have a severe allergy to the metal nickel that is commonly used as a base for plating of other metals. The rash may be localized to the ear lobes or to the area of the wrist under a watch, or to the abdominal area under a belt buckle. It will appear similar to the above eruptions in most cases.

Generalized Allergic Eruptions

A different kind of allergic dermatitis is the generalized eruption that is caused by becoming allergic to a substance that is taken internally or one that is introduced into the body by some sort of injection. That eruption is due to the body's immune system reacting to a foreign protein or other substance by forming antibodies. Those antibodies are circulated to every organ in the body, including the skin. Typical examples of those allergens are strawberries or shellfish or penicillin or iodine-containing compounds that can be given by injection or taken orally. The resultant rash is usually generalized over the entire body surface. It appears as redness with urticaria and is intensely itchy.

It should be mentioned that any allergic skin eruption might, in some individuals, simultaneously be accompanied by other serious forms of allergic response to the allergen. Those can include asthmatic wheezing and severe generalized collapse and even death as the body reacts violently to the allergen.

ERUPTIONS DUE TO VIRAL INFECTION

The rashes of viral infections are called viral exanthems. Childhood viral exanthems commonly include measles, German measles, chicken pox, and roseola infantum. The skin eruptions of exanthems are caused by the extension of the viral infection into the dermis. There an immunologic reaction occurs. The metabolic products of that immune reaction are responsible for the skin eruptions. The reactions due to various different viral infections cause skin eruptions of different characteristic appearance and distribution. Those differences enable us to identify the disease fairly easily.

All of the childhood exanthems carry the possibility of complications, chiefly due to the spread of the infection to other organs. The most feared of those complications is encephalitis (infection of the brain by the infecting virus.) Fortunately, the incidence of those complications is very low, but the knowledge of the danger enforces the need for having all children immunized against the common exanthems.

This chapter will be confined to the most commonly seen viral exanthems of children.

Roseola Infantum

Commonly called "roseola", this is a viral infection of infants. The incubation period is 5-15 days after exposure to the virus. The symptoms appear abruptly with high fever to 105 degrees F. and in some cases with convulsions caused by the high fever. That is a very frightening thing to the parents. The lymph nodes in the infant's neck usually become enlarged. A rash appears on the chest and abdomen and to a lesser degree on the face and extremities. The rash is called "maculo-papular" in medical parlance, meaning that it is flat or raised. It is pink to red in color, blotchy-rounded. The rash subsides in one to two days after its appearance and the fever then subsides. The disease is over in about a week from the time of onset of fever. There are usually no complications.

Chickenpox, (Varicella)

The incubation period after exposure is 14-16 days. The early eruptions are red macules, (flat or slightly raised spots) which first appear on the face, then extend outward to include the entire body and extremities. The macules then progress to become vesicles, (small blisters containing clear fluid). The infecting viruses actually are present in the fluid within the vesicles. The vesicles then dry to dry and become crusts. The patient remains contagious until the crusts all fall off, which usually is about three weeks after the onset of symptoms.

German Measles, (Rubella)

Rubella has an incubation period of 14-21 days after exposure. Low-grade fever and headache and fatigue are common during that time. The rash appears as blotchy red macules on the back of the neck and behind the ears. In those areas there is conspicuous enlargement of the lymph nodes that is a diagnostic sign of this disease. The rash extends to the face then to the extremities and trunk. The macules persist for about three days from the time of first appearance It then subsides, disappearing quickly.

Measles, (Rubeola)

Measles has an incubation period of 7-14 days after the first exposure. Symptoms begin with a hacking cough, usually accompanied by fever that may range from 101 to 105 degrees. 2-4 days later there is the appearance of Koplik spots, white irregular spots on the lining of the cheeks and on the tongue. A red, blotchy macular rash appears 3-5 days after the onset of fever, usually on the sides of the neck and in front and behind the ears, extending to the face and then to the trunk and extremities. There is usually fever of 104-105 degrees for several days more. The rash gradually changes to coppery brown, and then flakes off. Symptoms disappear about two weeks after the onset of the cough and fever.

The above are the most commonly seen viral exanthems. There are many others, some of minor importance and others that are often fatal, but they are too numerous and uncommonly seen in this country to be included in this text. The one most conspicuously known is smallpox, which we hope will remain on the list of "eradicated diseases." West Nile Fever however is now prevalent in the United States and threatens to become an epidemic. That disease is occasionally fatal. Information about exanthems seen in Africa and other countries is available from the Centers for Disease Control, (C.D.C.) on line. New emerging viral diseases are always present, and are quite frightening. The most notable of those are Ebola and Marburg disease. Avian Influenza (Bird Flu) is a new and potentially deadly epidemic infection that has been seen chiefly in Asia, but has made its appearance in Europe and in a very few cases in this country. It is a virus infection that is transmitted through infected poultry and wild birds. Only very recently has an immunizing vaccine been developed, and that is as yet untested and in an epidemic would be in very short supply. The World Health Organization is making great efforts to isolate the infected vectors and to destroy those birds.

Although this is not a textbook of pediatric medicine, there is one childhood disease that is frequently associated with measles and chickenpox and is included in routine immunizations. That is MUMPS. Even though that disease is not associated with an exanthematous rash I have chosen to include a brief description of mumps at this point.

Mumps (Epidemic Parotitis)

After a 12-24 day incubation period following exposure the symptoms begin with headache, low-grade fever, loss of appetite, and malaise. The patient may then begin to experience pain in the Parotid and Submandibular salivary glands upon tasting acidic, sour substances, such as lemon or vinegar. The Parotid salivary glands are located just in front and below the ears. The submandibular glands are located just medially to the angle of the jawbones, in the neck region. All four of those glands can be felt quite easily with some practice.

The salivary glands become very swollen and tender and the body temperature usually rises to about 104 degrees. Chewing and swallowing are painful. The swelling and fever usually subside within a week after appearance and recovery ensues.

The chief complication of mumps is involvement of the testicles with swelling, pain, and fever. This complication is called Orchitis. In most cases orchitis subsides with conservative treatment, but in some cases the outcome of this viral infection of the testes is permanent impairment of spermatogenesis, causing sterility. Mumps virus occasionally invades the pancreas, causing a serious pancreatitis. Fortunately, that life-threatening complication and mumps orchitis are extremely rare in childhood and the disease is usually quite mild.

As was stated at the beginning of the section of childhood viral exanthems, other complications are possible with any of these diseases, including encephalitis. These are major diseases with major complications. Immunization in infancy and early childhood can prevent them, in the great majority of cases and should absolutely be given to every child.

HERPES VIRUS INFECTIONS

In the preceding section we have discussed virus infections that cause childhood exanthems. There is another kind of virus infection that involves the skin, caused by viruses of the Herpes group. Herpes infections are common in people of all ages, but rarely in children. There are two distinct strains of viruses involved: the Herpes Simplex and the Herpes Zoster strains. They are different from each other and cause distinctly separate kinds of disease. We will begin with Herpes Simplex infections.

Herpes Simplex

Herpes simplex virus causes infections that are primarily in the skin, but can involve adjacent tissues also. There are two types of Herpes Simplex viruses called type A and type B. Type B Herpes is in most cases passed by genital contact from person to person and involves mainly the skin in the genital regions. Type A Herpes is seen in all other areas of the body. It must be stated, however, that there is some degree of crossover in the identification of the two viruses and the line of distinction between genital and non-genital Herpes is rather blurred.

Type A Herpes, the "non-genital" type can occur anywhere on the body surface. In many cases there is no recall or explanation of how the infection was contracted from another person. The lesions present as dusky red or pink macules with a clear vesicle, (blister), in the center. They are painful or itchy. They can last several days to weeks, then the vesicles dry and the macules fade away. It is very common for lesions to recur in the same areas at indeterminate times. That is because the virus continues to live within the dermis layer of the skin. There is no known means of curing and eradicating Herpes Simplex infections. There are effective antiviral medications to suppress the virus and to minimize the likelihood of recurrence, but as of the time of this writing there is no curative medication.

"Fever blisters" or "cold sores" on the lips are a form of Herpes Simplex infection. There is some evidence that the recurrence of the blisters is in part due to strong exposure to sunlight.

Type B or "genital Herpes" begins in much the same manner as type A. The lesions appear similar, but occur chiefly in the genital regions. In females there is a tendency for the lesions to occur on the mucosal surfaces of the vagina. That is not only painful, but carries an associated risk. There is an increased tendency in women who have genital Herpes to have cancer of the cervix if the lesions extend deeply within the vagina. It is not uncommon for vaginal lesions to be treated by some form of surgery to eradicate them as completely as possible.

Type B Herpes simplex can be treated with the same antiviral medications as type A, but is much more resistant to such treatment than is type A. There is good reason for concern when one party of a couple has this infection. Certainly, there should be no intercourse as long as any lesions are visible, but, in fact, there may be residual intravaginal lesions after most of the visible lesions have disappeared. The only protection against transmission of the disease is the use of condoms, or better yet, the avoidance of sexual contact for an adequate time after all lesions have disappeared. Unfortunately, "an adequate time" is a very elastic and indeterminate length of time for real safety.

Herpes Zoster

The virus bearing this name is a member of the Herpes family of viruses. Herpes zoster is thought to be caused by a reactivation of the same virus which caused Chicken Pox in childhood, then remained in a latent, inactive form in a sensory nerve cell, within the spinal chord. However, it manifests itself in an entirely different manner than Chicken Pox. The common name for this infection is "Shingles." For reasons that are entirely unclear the Herpes zoster virus has a propensity to infect only spinal nerve roots, and only the dorsal horns, or sensory part of the spinal nerve. Where an infected spinal nerve makes connection with a peripheral nerve the infecting virus also makes the connection and travels to the end of the line with that nerve, which is a sensory nerve ending in the skin.

Single sensory nerves can have many nerve endings in the skin. Sensory nerves are present in the skin in all parts of the body, including the head and face but Shingles occurs most commonly in the thoracic or abdominal regions. A nerve travels from the midline posteriorly to, but not beyond the midline anteriorly, giving off nerve endings to the surface of the skin all the way. The Herpes zoster virus travels with those nerve endings to the surface of the skin, and there establishes a lesion. The lesions are red macules with a vesicle in the center of each macule.

The resulting appearance is a red-to tan line of small blisters extending from the midline of the back to the midline of the chest, or abdomen. Because neither sensory nor motor nerves from the spine cross the midline anteriorly that is where the line of lesions stops. That is a very important fact in distinguishing Herpes zoster from some other types of skin eruptions.

Because the virus infects sensory nerves the lesions are extremely painful. Patients with this infection are often very difficult to manage because of the pain.

Herpes zoster does respond to treatment with antiviral medications, but is very resistant and slow to heal. The pain is so severe that strong analgesic medications are required, often needing narcotics to make the patient comfortable. In cases of prolonged duration there is some danger of creating addiction to the analgesic medication. An expensive preventive vaccine has become available and is recommended for aged individuals

There is a phenomenon called Post-Herpetic Pain. In patients with that diagnosis the severe pain of the Herpes zoster lesions persists after all evidence of skin lesions has subsided. That is a complicated problem, usually requiring consultation with pain management specialists and neurologic and often psychiatric specialists.

There is a specific complication of Herpes zoster that was discussed in the chapter on eye disorders, but bears repetition here. In cases where the infected nerve is a facial nerve a branch can travel to the forehead and face, sending a sensory branch to the cornea of the eye. In the event that Herpes zoster lesions appear on the cornea there can be extensive scar formation on the cornea. In some cases the scarring can be so severe and extensive as to cause complete opacification of the cornea. For that reason, any Herpes zoster infection of the eye must be treated by a competent ophthalmologist, as soon as possible, in order to avoid the prospect of needing corneal transplant surgery, or incurring blindness in that eye.

BACTERIAL INFECTIONS OF THE SKIN

The most common skin infection due to bacteria is the secondary infection of injuries to the skin. Most infections due to accidental injury, if involving only the skin, can be assumed to be due to a commonly occurring bacterial organism, probably susceptible to commonly used medications. They are usually best treated with careful cleansing of the wound and possibly the use of topical antibiotic ointments or creams. If the wound becomes red or drainage occurs medical attention should be obtained. That is best because in some instances the infection can be caused by an extremely aggressive and resistant organism and might require special treatment, possibly including hospital care.

The infection of a surgically sustained wound is another kind of problem. The question arises as to how the wound became infected and if a resistant organism is responsible. Doctors take those infections very seriously because of the possibility of a resistant bacterium being the cause. They are also most interested in the explanation of how and why the surgical wound became infected. Never hesitate to consult your doctor immediately if signs of an infection occur. The concern of hospital-acquired infections occurring during the operation or in the recovery period is always present in the mind or a surgeon.

Pimples, Blackheads, Whiteheads

Of course, those terms are too simple for doctors to use. The medical term for pimples is "pustules", and for blackheads "comedones." They are closely related. A whitehead is a blocked oil duct, covered by a thin layer of epidermis showing through the surface of the skin. A blackhead or comedone is the dark collection of oil that has plugged the duct of an oil gland and has become unroofed, allowing the oxygen of the air to oxidize the oil, changing it to a dark pigment. A pimple or pustule is a bacterial infection in a plugged duct of an oil gland. These can occur at any age, but most often plague the lives of teen-agers. Boils, (furuncles), are very large versions of pimples. They are usually more deeply situated in the skin layers and are almost always due to Staphyllococcal infection. Furuncles frequently have multiple "heads", presenting on the surface of the skin. Because of the large size and depth of the infection they are usually painful. In all cases of repeated appearance of furuncles or the appearance of multiple furuncles at one time, a medical consultation is advisable to consider the possibility of some condition that would reduce the patient's resistance to such infections. Surgical drainage of furuncles is frequently required.

Acne

That is the name given to an extremely common skin problem that is most commonly, but certainly not exclusively, seen in adolescents. The hormonal changes of adolescence produce a copious thick secretion of oil from the sebaceous glands of the skin. This is not true in every adolescent, but does affect most of teenage boys, and to a lesser degree, girls. The infection in acne is almost always a Staphyllococcal bacterium. "Staph." infections used to be easy to treat with penicillin and other common antibiotics. However, in recent years many strains of Staph have become resistant to many antibiotics. The cornerstone of acne treatment is common sense skin care. Washing with mild soap, the avoidance of hard scrubbing that would injure the skin and the application of mild lotions and potions that are antibacterial and mildly drying. Diet does not seem to make much difference. Any medication that feels painful upon application is bad and should be avoided. A moderate amount of sun exposure is good, but serious sunburn should be avoided. If the pustules and comedones are too much to manage at home, see your primary care doctor or a dermatologist. Antibiotic medication may be required for the severe cases.

The most severe complication of acne is the residual scarring that it frequently causes, in spite of the best treatment. Severe cases of acne usually cause permanent thickening and scarring. This is most often seen on the back where the skin is thicker, but scarring is also quite common on the face. In cases where the scarring is extensive and severe, there is no practical treatment to restore a state of cosmetic normalcy. There are, however, many dermatologists who specialize in acne restoration and it is worthwhile to have such a consultation.

SEVERE BACTERIAL INFECTIONS OF THE SKIN

There are a number of severe bacterial infections that involve the skin. Many deserve in-depth discussion, but for the purposes of this text we will cover only the two most commonly seen.

Impetigo

Impetigo is an acute bacterial infection of the skin that is transmitted from person to person by contact. It is most commonly seen in children of early school age. The causative organ is a Staphyllococcus bacterium.

The first sign of an impetigo infection is a slightly raised patch of buff-to red skin. That patch then ulcerates, leaving a wet crater exuding pus. The exudate contains living bacteria that can then colonize, spreading the infection. The extent of affected skin can be quite large if treatment is not instituted promptly. Permanent scarring can result.

Impetigo can usually be arrested and cured by antibiotic therapy. It is imperative that good skin care be given at home, with frequent gentle cleansing. Your primary care physician should be contacted at the first sign of the typical eruptions.

Hydradenitis Suppurativa

In some individuals the axillary apocrine sweat glands have an unusual susceptibility to become infected with bacteria. It may be due to the increased viscosity of their secretions plugging the ducts through which the secretions pass. The translation of the name into English means "Infection of fluid-secreting glands due to pus-forming bacteria".

When infected, those glands that are normally microscopic in size fill with pus, becoming abscesses, and enlarging to the size of a pea, or greater. As the infection spreads the surrounding skin becomes very red and the pain can be severe. It is usually necessary to drain the abscessed glands surgically and to prescribe antibiotic medications.

Hydradenitis Suppurativa infections usually do not begin before adulthood. Once they begin they have a tendency to recur and to become progressively more severe. It is not unusual for people afflicted with this disorder to require extensive surgical removal of all the sweat, and apocrine glands in the axillae. Fortunately, this infection does not seem to occur in the peri-anal apocrine glands.

FUNGAL INFECTIONS OF THE SKIN

The general medical name given to fungal infections of the skin is "dermatophytoses", because the type of fungal organisms that cause skin infections are called "Dermatophytes". Also included under this heading are fungus infections of the nails. Fungus organisms are in our environment virtually at all times universally. They grow best in conditions of heat and moisture and many do best in darkness, rather than in light. In tropical climates it is not unusual for fungus infections to occur on the skin of any part of the body. In most non-tropical environments the most common sites of fungus infections are the feet, between the toes because of the conditions of warmth, moisture and darkness within most shoes. The skin folds of the body, such as groins, armpits, and the skin folds beneath the breasts are also common sites of fungus infections, for the same reasons, especially in warm conditions.

Individual susceptibility to fungus infections varies greatly. It is uncommon for most people living in temperate climates to have dermatophyte infections of exposed areas of the skin. There is usually an explanation having to do with individual susceptibility, such as being diabetic, or having a disease that causes an immunocompromised state, such as HIV infection or leukemia, or being exposed to conditions of heat and moisture for long periods of time. In such cases fungus infections of the toenails or skin are often seen. In hot, humid tropical climates one is much more likely to have dermatophytosis of the skin or fingernails.

Fungus infections of the feet and toenails are very common in all climatic conditions as the result of wearing shoes. Men are much more susceptible because their shoes are usually much more enclosing than are women's shoes. Skin infections of the foot and toes are commonly called "Athlete's Foot". Those infections are usually easily managed with simple topical medications and skin care.

Fungus infections of the nails are called "Onychomycosis" in Doctor Speak (meaning, fungus infections of the nails). Even though there are many remedies for fungus infections of the toenails, in most men there is a disturbing tendency for the infection to subside with treatment, then to return. Although most people, and with good cause, look for a cure, probably the most reasonable solution to the problem is to apply topical medications to the skin and toenails in order to keep the infection minimal, but not to expect a cure.

A very common site for dermatophytosis, called Tinea Cruris in medical terminology, is the crural region, that area including the groins and the scrotum in men. The skin of the crural region fulfills the criteria of being warm, moist, and dark. In men it is commonly called "jock itch" because it is most likely, but not exclusively, to occur in men who exercise and sweat more than others. The best treatment for that condition is good personal hygiene, frequent bathing, and the application of ant fungal cream or gel as needed.

There are many more fungus infections of the skin. Some of those seen in the tropics are very severe. This chapter will discuss only one more very common fungal infection; Tinea Versicolor.

Tinea Versicolor

This infection is most common in warm climates where there is a tendency to sweat. The fungal growth is seen mainly on the skin of the back and shoulders and to a lesser extent on the front of the chest and the abdomen. The fungus organism that causes this infection invades the skin and extends through the epidermis into the dermal layer. There it invades the pigment-forming cells, reducing their ability to manufacture pigment. As a result, during the summer when we expose our bodies to the sun, there is failure of the skin to tan evenly. This causes a mottling of the skin, with the unaffected cells tanning normally and the infected cells appearing pale. When we are not exposed to the sun the tan fades and the infected cells give the skin a buff, or mildly tan appearance.

Tinea versicolor is very widely prevalent in areas of warm climate. There is effective treatment in the form of topically applied medications that can be prescribed by your primary care physician. Dermatologist consultation may not be necessary. Some individuals who have greater susceptibility than most experience recurrence of the infection and require periodic treatment. There are no serious systemic complications.

The dark skin of people of African descent behaves differently when infected with Tinea Versicolor. The infected cells become more intensely pigmented, causing ragged areas of darker pigmentation. That discoloration remains until the infection is cured.

INSECT INFESTATIONS

Insect infestations are very commonly seen in animals, such as monkeys and other primates. The two most frequently seen in humans are pediculosis, which means infestations by lice, and scabies, which is skin infestation by mites. Both are very common in our society.

Pediculosis

There are two kinds of louse infections in humans: head and body. Head lice are very frequently seen in young children. The infestation is spread by contact, usually while in kindergarten or the early grades of school. Itching of the scalp is the only symptom. Examination of the head reveals the presence of small crawling insects and the presence of their eggs which are attached to the bases of hairs. The eggs are within small sacs that are called nits.

Treatment consists of the eradication of as many lice as possible by brushing and combing the hair and the application of solutions that are toxic to the lice, but not to humans. Prophylactic treatment of every child in the class is strongly recommended to stop further passage of the infestation. Your primary care physician can advise the best medication currently available.

Body lice, commonly called "crabs", are usually seen in the pubic region. The only symptom is itching in that region. The insects can be seen crawling on the skin of the pubic area and the abdomen. Their eggs can be seen in sacs adhering to the pubic hairs. Transmission can be by two routes: direct contact from body-to-body and by using a bed, the linens of which were not changed after being used by someone with a louse infestation.

Treatment is the same as that used for eradication of head lice. It is strongly recommended that for either infestation the application of medication be repeated four days after the initial application to kill the lice that might have hatched in the intervening time.

Scabies

This is a skin infestation caused by a mite, a smaller insect than the louse. The symptom is intense itching of the affected areas of the body. The mode of transmission is the same as that of pediculosis; either bodily contact, or from bedding in which the mite was present. The diagnosis is more difficult than that of pediculosis. Tiny red spots can be seen on the skin, representing the entrance to burrows made by the mites. For a positive diagnosis it is frequently necessary to open the burrow with a small instrument and to extract the mite for microscopic examination.

Treatment is the same as that for pediculosis. Whenever possible it is advisable to trace back to the source of the infestation in order to limit further communication of the infection.

INFLAMMATORY DISORDERS OF THE SKIN

Rosacea

This is a chronic disorder, cause unknown. It is characterized by redness, proliferation of small blood vessels in the skin and thickening of the skin resembling orange peel texture. It is most often seen on the nose, the adjacent skin and forehead. It is most often seen in people with fair complexion, usually beginning in the early forties and continuing as a chronic disorder, often for the lifetime. There is no known relationship to diet, or to alcohol intake, although it is a very common misconception that people who have rosacea are chronic alcoholics.

There is no known curative treatment. Consultation with a dermatologist is recommended for the best guidance and treatment.

Eczema

This is a skin eruption that can occur at any age. The cause is unknown, but there has been association with allergy and with emotional stress.

The eruption can vary from a few small patches of rounded or oval pink with white scaling at the edges to involvement of most of the body. There is often associated itching. The eruptions can occur suddenly and then clear, only to recur again. The course can be brief or chronic.

Treatment is directed at relieving the itching and suppressing the progress of the eruptions. Corticosteroid medication is often very helpful. It is best to share the care with your primary care physician or with a dermatologist for best results.

Psoriasis

This is a skin eruption that is clearly immunologic in origin. It is associated with a type of arthritis called Psoriatic Arthritis. Psoriasis can show its first manifestations early in life and last a lifetime. Early eruptions have pink centers with white scaly edges. The eruptions frequently do not clear, but remain, enlarging with time. It is not unusual for most of the back and sides of the trunk to be involved. There is no associated itching.

Psoriasis is clearly a skin eruption that should be managed by a physician because of the associated arthritis and the chronicity of the disorder.

SKIN CYSTS

Cysts can occur anywhere in the body. They are hollow structures that contain the product of the tissue of origin. Thus breast cysts contain the fluid produced by the breast glands, and thyroid cysts contain the product of the thyroid gland. Skin cysts are technically called "Epidermal Inclusion cysts", meaning that they present on the surface of the skin and contain some product of the glands that are located in that area of the skin.

The most commonly seen skin cysts are sebaceous cysts. The name implies that they arise from oil (sebaceous) glands. The glands that produce skin oil are situated in the dermis layer of the skin. The oil that they produce is carried through small ducts to the surface of the skin to lubricate the skin. If a pore through which the oil exits from the duct becomes plugged by dried and thickened oil it becomes a blackhead, (comedone). If the duct remains blocked the gland will continue to manufacture oil, but it will not be able to exit from the gland. The gland, which in its native state is of microscopic size, enlarges to many times its original size. At first it is a barely noticeable bump on the skin, bur it continues to enlarge, sometimes to tremendous size if untreated. I have seen sebaceous cysts the size of golf balls in my practice.

The oil that is produced by the sebaceous glands is thin and clear in its native state. When the duct becomes blocked it begins to dry and thicken. If a blackhead is squeezed, and blackhead will pop out, and with it a thin ribbon of cheesy substance that smells sour and rancid. That is called sebum, the contents of the sebaceous cyst.

If the cyst continues to enlarge, the only good treatment is to have it removed surgically. That is usually a simple procedure in your doctor's office, or that of a dermatologist. Larger cysts involve greater difficulty in removal and should be removed only by an experienced surgeon.

TUMORS OF THE SKIN—BENIGN TUMORS

Fibromas

Fibromas are among the most common of skin tumors. They are derived from fibrous elements of the epidermis. They have no single characteristic appearance. They are usually lightly pigmented and can be in any location on the skin. They can vary from small dots to linear streaks to large patches of leathery appearance. Fibromas may also present as fleshy growths on the end of thin stalks of skin. They do not have a tendency to become malignant, but will in most cases enlarge if left alone. In prominent locations they are often considered to be unsightly.

Fibromas are usually very easily removed under local anesthesia in a doctor's office.

Lipomas

Lipomas are the most common of benign skin tumors. They are composed of mature yellow fat cells encased in a sac of connective tissue. They usually grow from the subcutaneous fat just deep to the dermal layer, and as they enlarge they push up the overlying skin, thinning it out. Lipomas can also grow from the deeper portion of the subcutaneous fat. They can vary greatly in size. They are soft to touch and are not tender or fluctuant to finger pressure.

Because they can grow to a huge size, it is best to have lipomas removed if they are in conspicuous or sensitive locations. Some lipomas become so large as to require a hospital-type surgery for removal, but most small lipomas can be removed under local anesthesia in a doctor's office.

Pigmented Nevi

These are commonly occurring benign skin growths. They appear as areas of pigmentation, usually in shades of brown to black, and in some cases they have a bluish appearance. They can occur in any location. They are usually flat, but can be slightly elevated and can be of any size, although it is very unusual to find a pigmented nevus greater than a centimeter in diameter. They are harmless benign growths. On a lady's face they are often referred to as "beauty marks".

The one precaution is that there is an extremely malignant skin tumor called MELANOMA that is pigmented and can have elements of brown, blue, or black pigment. It is wise to have a physician or dermatologist check any pigmented skin tumor to rule out that cancer. Melanomas will be discussed in more detail in the section on malignant skin tumors.

Keratoses

Keratoses are quite common after the age of forty. The cause for their occurrence is unknown. They are firm growths of the superficial epithelial layer of the skin, containing keratin. They are most commonly pigmented, having a tan to brown appearance. They can be horny projections or linear streaks or firm clumps. Keratoses most commonly occur on the trunk, favoring the back, but are also quite common on the face and eyelids.

Keratoses are in most cases benign, but may occasionally have a malignant potential. Most Keratoses can be removed as an office surgical procedure.

Hemangiomas

Hemangiomas are tumors that are composed of masses of blood vessels just within the surface of the epidermis. The blood vessels originate in the dermis layer, but because of their size they present on the surface of the skin. When they appear as a web-like pink or red blotch on the skin they are called capillary hemangiomas, because they are composed of many capillaries. Larger and more deeply red hemangiomas are called cavernous hemangiomas, because they actually are composed of a pool of blood within the skin. Both capillary and cavernous hemangiomas are congenital in origin.

Both capillary and cavernous hemangiomas are quite often extremely difficult to remove because in the required surgery the damage to the underlying skin could be quite extensive. They can be extremely large, even covering most of one half of the patient's face. In such cases it is often the best judgment to leave it untreated, because of the possible damage inflicted by the treatment.

There is a class of hemangiomas that are acquired, rather than congenital in origin. These are called "spider angiomas." They are usually seen on the skin of the legs. They are much more common in women than in men.

Spider angiomas are formed by an arteriole in the dermis emptying into a network of capillaries and causing the capillaries to enlarge visibly, just under the surface of the skin.

Spider angiomas can be diagnosed by applying pressure over the network of vessels, then releasing the pressure. With the application of pressure the vessels empty, and that area of skin appears pale. When the pressure is released the capillaries immediately fill again, from the center outward.

Spider angiomas do not cause any health problems but can appear unsightly on a lady's leg. They can be removed by laser treatment, usually by a dermatologist. There is some risk of residual scar formation by that treatment.

MALIGNANT TUMORS OF THE SKIN

Basal Cell Carcinoma

These are the most commonly seen skin cancers. They grow from the basal cell layer of the epidermis. They can occur anywhere on the body's surface. They are technically a cancer because if untreated they continue to grow larger and deeper, ultimately requiring extensive surgical removal. They do not metastasize to distant sites or organs as do some other cancers.

A typical basal cell carcinoma appears as a flat, round change in the superficial skin with a buff-colored to pink smooth surface and edges that appear slightly rolled. The growth of the tumor occurs at its edges. They are not very deep initially and are painless and nontender. In time the center of the tumor may appear slightly depressed.

In most cases scraping the surface and burning the area of the tumor with an electric cautery needle can remove a basal cell carcinoma. Although this treatment is very commonly employed it does leave some concern that the cancer has not been completely removed. That is especially true if the cancer is on the face, because if some tumor is inadvertently left in place the remaining tumor will grow larger and deeper, requiring more extensive surgery at a later time.

In most cases I recommend a surgical excision under local anesthesia, taking a good margin of normal skin around and beneath the tumor. That requires suturing the wound, but it is the most positive way of curing the cancer. If sutured skillfully the resultant scar will be, in most cases, less conspicuous than if the scrape and burn technique is used.

Squamous Cell Carcinoma

These cancers also arise from the basal layer of the epidermis. They are most often found on the lips and nose, although they can occur in other areas of the skin. They tend to be flat and thin, with scaly or flaky edges. They also enlarge by spreading and growing deeper into the skin if untreated. This cancer has, in some cases, the potential to metastasize to different areas and organs of the body. That fact greatly increases its potential danger. Squamous cell carcinomas certainly should be removed by wide and deep surgical excision. Treatment should never be by scraping and burning the lesion.

Melanoma

Melanomas are the most malignant of all skin cancers. They actually rank among the most malignant of all cancers in the body. They arise from the basal cell layer of the epidermis from cells that produce melanin pigment. They are given that name because of the presence of melanin pigment in most melanomas. You may recall that melanin pigment is responsible for the color of the skin, the iris of the eye, and the hair. Depending on the concentration and intensity of the pigment in the tumor melanomas can vary in color from brown to blue-gray to jet black. There is a type of melanoma called "amelanotic melanoma" that lacks the typical pigment of melanoma and can be diagnosed only by microscopic examination. That fact reinforces the need for excision of all skin tumors in order to obtain a biopsy for microscopic examination by a competent pathologist, and possibly to be cured in their earliest stages.

Melanomas are most commonly seen in people with fair skin, blond or red hair, and often in those with a tendency to freckle formation. They can arise in any area of the skin, but are by far the most common in skin that is exposed to prolonged and intense sunlight. In recent years there has been an epidemic of melanomas in areas where the sun is the most intense, and people are exposing their bodies more in water sports. There is also a definite familial incidence of melanoma.

Melanoma has a very strong tendency to metastasize through the lymphatic and blood vessels. Metastatic cells can be found in the regional lymph nodes closest to the original skin tumor due to extension via the lymphatic vessels. Metastasis rarely occurs to remote areas, such as bone or brain due to travel via the blood vessels. Melanoma is a highly aggressive cancer and often results in death.

In each case; basal cell, squamous cell cancers, or melanoma, the cancer is first evidenced by a visible change on the skin. This means that in the earliest stages those cancers are usually curable. Melanoma is somewhat of an exception to that rule because of its tendency to metastasize before it becomes evident on the skin. The point of this comment is that in the case of most skin cancers there is a possibility of cure in the earliest stage of the disease, if it is discovered early. Any persistent change on the surface of the skin should be reported to your doctor or to a dermatologist. It is in this case that there is wisdom to the old adage, "when in doubt, take it out" so that the tumor can be examined and adequate care be given as early as possible.

Chapter Ten
THE MUSCULOSKELETAL SYSTEM

Although they are very different tissues the muscles and bones are very closely related functionally and both will be discussed in this chapter, in addition to tendons and ligaments.

MUSCLES

Muscles make the body move. Every system of the body in which movement is part of its function depends on some sort of muscle activity.

There are two kinds of muscles: those that make our arms, legs, and large body areas move are called the "voluntary" muscles. The muscles that work without our knowledge, making the cardio-vascular, digestive, and urinary-gynecologic systems function are called the "involuntary" muscles. Some organs of the body depend on a combination of both types of muscles for their normal functioning.

Although they both function by making parts move, the voluntary and involuntary muscles are quite different in microscopic appearance and nerve supply. The Voluntary muscles when seen under the microscope have lines that traverse their width at very close intervals. Because of that they are called "striated" muscles, ("striations" means streaks, or lines). They receive their nerve stimulus from the "voluntary" nervous system-that which we control volitionally. The Involuntary muscles do not contain striations, and are called "smooth" muscles. They are supplied with nerves from the autonomic or "involuntary" nervous system. The muscle of which the heart is composed is a special kind of smooth muscle and receives its nerve stimulation from the autonomic nervous system and its own built-in pacemaker and conduction system.

These are complicated concepts on the surface, but they get simpler when you understand that the big "muscles" that we see on the surface of the body are striated muscle, and the invisible muscles that cause the peristalsis that moves food through the digestive tract, and the muscles that widen or narrow the pupil of the eye are smooth muscles.

We should take a few minutes to examine just what makes muscles move. The basic principle is much the same as that in how we see and how we hear. Every muscle is supplied with nerves; sensory nerves that tell the brain how it feels and motor nerves that tell the muscle to move. The means by which nerves stimulate muscles to contract, and muscles send sensory impulses to the nerves to be forwarded to the brain is by synaptic transfer of electrical stimuli, in which there is the chemical reaction that occurs with acetylcholine, between nerve and muscle.

All muscle movement is a matter of contraction of the muscle fibers, followed by relaxation of those fibers. When a motor nerve of either the voluntary or involuntary system sends its signal to its appropriate muscle a chemical reaction occurs within each muscle cell. Compounds within the muscle cell break down, releasing minute amounts of electrical energy. The muscle fiber, fueled mainly by sugar and oxygen, then contracts.

When millions of muscle cells contract at once the muscle shortens, causing an arm or a finger or the tongue to move. Then the muscle relaxes, releasing carbon dioxide and the products of sugar metabolism, chiefly lactic acid, into the blood stream to be further metabolized. That, in a very much shortened and simplified manner, is how the engine of the muscles works.

TENDONS AND LIGAMENTS

Muscles attach to bones and to the other body parts that they cause to move by means of tendons. Tendons are composed of fibrous tissue, usually with some elastic characteristic. They can be thick, massive, and very strong, such as the Achilles tendon that attaches the calf muscles to the bone of the heel, or very small and fragile, such as the tendons that attach muscles to the eyelids. Tendons are living tissue, with blood and nerve supply. They metabolize, using oxygen and nutrients, and they create waste products that have to be taken away by the blood stream.

Ligaments are strong fibrous straps or bands that attach bones to bones or, in some cases, parts of the body to adjacent parts. They also can be massive or very small and they are living tissues that have a blood and nerve supply, require oxygen and nutrients, and they create waste products, as do other tissues.

FASCIA

Fascia is the name given to all fibrous connective tissue throughout the body. It varies in size and thickness, but is generally found in sheets that enclose muscle bundles and give shape to the muscles. Fascia can serve to attach muscles to bone, but most commonly lends strength and form to large areas of the body, such as the abdomen and the extremities. A good example of fascia that can be felt easily is the lateral areas of the thighs, where the muscles are encased in a thick, strong sheet of fascia, called the "fascia lata" that forms the flat surface of the side of the thigh.

DISORDERS OF THE MUSCLES AND TENDONS

Muscles can rupture. In many cases a muscle rupture can be seen on the surface of the body. Rupture of a skeletal muscle is a very common problem. It is actually a muscle coming apart, usually as in the case of a very heavy strain placed on a previously injured muscle. Muscle rupture is manifested by pain, local swelling, and, frequently, bleeding, visible as bruising of the skin. The part of the body that depends on that muscle for movement moves only partially and with severe pain, or not at all. In most cases the muscle can be repaired surgically.

A very commonly seen muscle rupture is that of the plantaris muscle in the calf of the leg. It is the result of a previously injured muscle coming apart when placed under minimal strain. The patient feels a minor popping sensation in the back of the leg, at mid-calf level, usually while bending forward. Upon examination there is a ridge extending across the middle of the calf. There is usually only mild tenderness. The plantaris is a thin muscle, serving only an auxiliary function, and so the leg continues to function fairly normally. The usual treatment is "calculated neglect", because the surgical repair would be very difficult, and the loss of that muscle causes only minimal dysfunction.

There are other kinds of muscle rupture that are not visible on the surface. One of the most serious of those is rupture of a papillary muscle within the heart. The papillary muscles are those that cause the valves of the heart to open. They originate in the muscle wall of the heart, and are connected to the valves by small tendons, called "chordae tendinae." When a papillary muscle ruptures or one of the chordae tendinae comes loose that heart valve fails to open. The result can be sudden death or severe cardiac dysfunction. That problem is remediable by means of open- heart surgery, usually done as an emergency.

Tendon rupture is quite common in men. The most commonly involved tendons are the Achilles tendon, connecting the gastrocnemius muscle of the calf to the heel bone, and rupture of the tendon of the long head of the biceps muscle, which normally extends from the shoulder to the forearm just below the elbow. Those muscles are very important in walking and lifting and pulling, respectively. They get much heavy use in many men. At some point in time, because of previous injury plus wear and tear, those tendons can rupture. When that happens, in the case of the Achilles tendon the muscle rolls up like a window shade, leaving a hollow depression in the lower leg and a roll of muscle in the mid-calf. In the case of the biceps tendon the muscle rolls down from the shoulder, leaving a hollow in the upper arm, and forming a roll of muscle in the middle of the upper arm. Achilles tendon rupture must be repaired as soon as possible because walking normally is dependent on an intact gastrocnemius-Achilles tendon connection in order to raise and plant the heel. The biceps muscle in the upper arm can function with only the short head tendon intact. Therefore it is not essential to repair a rupture of the tendon of the long head in most cases.

Those two examples were given as illustrations of the relationship between muscles and tendons, and how such injuries are commonly managed medically.

Hernias

An abdominal hernia is defined as the protrusion of a loop or a knuckle of an organ or tissue through an abnormal opening in the abdomen. The most common example of that term is a muscle weakness that is visible and palpable on the surface of the abdomen with protrusion through the weakness. There is another kind of hernia that is very serious. That is an internal hernia within the abdomen. That kind of hernia was discussed at length in the chapter on the digestive system.

Another kind of hernia is that of severe weakness and widening of the opening in the diaphragm through which the esophagus passes to connect with the stomach. The esophageal hiatus hernia was also discussed at length in the chapter on the digestive system. By far the most commonly occurring hernias are abdominal hernias called "inguinal hernias", involving the muscles and fascia in the groin, either leading to the scrotum or presenting anteriorly in the low abdomen as a bulge. Hernias that extend through the inguinal ligament and extend toward, or enter the scrotum are called "Indirect Inguinal Hernias." Those presenting anteriorly on the abdominal surface are called "Direct Inguinal Hernias." Another very common type of hernia is the "ventral hernia", involving the mid or upper abdominal muscle and fascial wall.

All of those hernias can be complicated by incarceration, (getting stuck in the hernial defect) of subcutaneous fat, or by incarceration of intestine or stomach. If the opening of the hernia is so tight as to interfere with the blood supply of the incarcerated tissue the hernia is called a "strangulated hernia." That is a condition that requires emergency surgery to release the incarcerated tissue before it dies.

In most cases hernias present as a weakness in the wall of the abdomen with a protruding lump coming from within the abdomen. The weakness and the lump are seen in either groin region, or in the mid or upper abdomen on one side or other of the midline. A variation of those hernias is the "umbilical hernia", in which the weakness is in the base of the umbilicus, ("belly button"). All of those abdominal hernias require surgical repair. That surgery can become an emergency if the hernia contains stomach, intestine, or other vital structures.

OTHER DISORDERS AFFECTING MUSCLE

Neuro-Muscular Diseases

The muscles of the body are remarkably free of general systemic diseases, but can be involved in a number of specific disorders. Some of those are due to the close relationship between muscle and the nervous system. There are a number of muscular dystrophies that cause progressive muscle weakness, incoordination, muscle wasting, and paralysis. One example of that group of diseases is "Lou Gehrig's disease", known in abbreviation as ALS. These are very complex disorders, requiring extensive diagnostic workups and specialized care. It is very important that in any person, at any age, a change in muscle strength, coordination, gait, or fine control deserves a good medical evaluation by competent physicians.

Myasthenia Gravis

This disease causes the inability of nerve cells to manufacture a substance called acetylcholine that is necessary for neuromuscular function. The cause is an auto-immune disorder. The symptoms can begin at any age, but are most often seen between the ages of 20 and 40. The earliest sign of this disorder is often drooping of the eyelids, (ptosis). Muscle weakness of the eyes is among the widespread forms of this disease. Severe muscle weakness and wasting are seen in a number of primarily neurologic disorders. Probably the one most frequently seen is multiple sclerosis. That disease was discussed at length in the chapter on the nervous system.

Poliomyelitis

This is a viral infection of the nervous system that has in the past been a major cause of permanent muscle wasting and loss of function, even causing paralysis of the muscles of respiration. Fortunately, that disease is now very rare, due to widespread immunization against the poliovirus.

Tumors of Muscles

Tumors can occur in muscles just as they can in any other tissue of the body. They are quite uncommon and unfortunately, many tumors of muscle are malignant. Soft tissue cancers other than those of muscles are called sarcomas. Cancers of muscle tissues are called leiomyosarcomas or rhabdomyosarcomas, depending on whether they originate in smooth or striated muscle. Such cancers can occur in muscle tissue anywhere in the body. The only worthwhile comment to the reader is to seek medical advice at the first appearance of any unusual and unexplained sign of growth or weakness in any muscle.

THE BONES—THE ANATOMY AND PHYSIOLOGY OF BONES

Bones are living tissue. They require oxygen and nutrients the same as all other tissues and produce carbon dioxide and the waste products of their metabolism. They grow and stop growing when stimulated by hormones from the pituitary gland.

There are two kinds of bone: the long bones, such as those in the extremities, and the flat bones, such as those in the skull, pelvis and vertebral column. The long bones have a thick, strong outer layer called the cortex and an inner network of thin bone, called cancellous bone. All bone is composed of calcium carbonate and calcium phosphate and other minerals, held together in a matrix of protein. The flat bones have a thin outer layer of dense cortical bone, and a spacious inner network of cancellous bone.

Bones do not have true blood vessels. Instead, they are pierced by small channels called canaliculi. Through those tiny channels blood cells penetrate the bone and provide for its nutrition and removal of waste products. On the outside of every bone is a thin, clear sheet of tissue called the periosteum, which is closely adherent to the bony cortex. Within the periosteum are blood vessels and nerves that ultimately connect with the canaliculi to supply the interior of the bones with those vital components.

A very good way to actually see the periosteum and its relationship to bone is to examine a spare rib the next time you are eating one. The thin sheet surrounding the bone is the periosteum.

Within the cancellous interior of all bone is the marrow space where red blood cells and some white blood cells are manufactured.

The growth of bone occurs at an area that is close to the ends of long bones, and around the edges of the flat bones. The growth centers of bones are called "the epiphyses." Bone growth goes on at those locations from the time of birth under the stimulus of growth hormone from the pituitary gland. The growth of bone stops when growth hormone production by the pituitary stops at some variable age. In most people that is before the age of thirty. Problems of growth hormone production and effect include very small stature due to under-production of the hormone and gigantism and acromegaly due to overproduction. Acromegaly is the abnormality in which there is marked enlargement of the head and jaw, as well as in the skeleton generally that is seen in cases of overproduction of growth hormone due to a tumor of the pituitary gland occurring after the normal cessation of growth hormone production.

THE ANATOMY OF THE SKELETON

The skeleton can be divided into two components: the axial skeleton, including the skull, the sternum, the long bones and the vertebral column, and the appendicular skeleton, including the ribs, the shoulder girdle, and the pelvis. For the purposes of this text we will describe the skeleton from the head downward, beginning with the skull.

In the interest of practicality and because this is not a textbook of anatomy the descriptions of each component will be sparse, but hopefully giving sufficient and useful information.

The Skull

Composed of several flat plates of bone, the skull of a newborn has many gaps to allow for growth. Those gaps fill in by age four or five, at which time the skull becomes a helmet, enclosing and protecting the most vital of all organs, the brain.

The skull has concave areas in its frontal region that are the orbits that contain the eyes. There are openings in the rear of the orbits for the optic nerves to travel to the brain. The nasal bones are the framework for the nose. There are four pairs of cavernous open spaces that contain the sinuses; the maxillary sinuses below the orbits, the frontal sinuses above the orbits, and the ethmoid and sphenoid sinuses below the space reserved for the brain. On each side of the skull there are openings for the ears, and on either side are the temporal bones that house the internal structures for hearing and equilibrium.

The mouth is formed by the maxilla, which is a dense solid ridge of bone beneath the maxillary sinuses, and the mandible. The mandible is a separate U-shaped bone that is closed in front and open at its rear edges. There it is hinged on either side by ligaments that attach it to the skull. Very strong muscles enable the mandible to open and to close with great force.

The skull is pierced by many openings that allow the passages of nerves and blood vessels. At the lower rear of the skull is a large opening called the occipital foramen, or foramen magnum that is the passage through which the spinal cord leaves the skull and enters the spinal canal. At that point the skull connects with the vertebral column.

The Vertebral Column

Commonly called "the spine", the vertebral column is a chain of cancellous bones that extends from the base of the skull to the "tailbone." The vertebral bones are held together by a series of very strong ligaments. Extending posteriorly from each vertebral body is a series of interconnecting bony arches that form a tunnel through which passes the spinal cord. The spinal cord is composed of very long tracts of nerve tissue. At each level of the vertebral column spinal nerves emerge on each side through openings called the foramina. At those points the nerves leave the central nervous system and become part or the peripheral nervous system. Peripheral nerves from the entire body, carrying messages to the central nervous system enter the vertebral column at the same levels.

The vertebral column is divided into three regional sections. In the region of the neck is the "cervical region" it is called the cervical spine, composed of seven cervical vertebrae. In the region of the chest, (the "thorax") it is called the thoracic spine. It contains twelve vertebrae extending from the base of the neck to the bottom of the chest, and in the low back, (the "lumbar region") it is called the lumbar spine, containing five vertebrae.

At the bottom of the fifth lumbar vertebra there is a long shield-shaped bone called the sacrum. Connected to the sacrum in four fused sections are the bones called the coccyx, commonly called "the tail-bone".

The Bones of the Chest

The ribs that form the framework of the chest begin in most people at the level of the first thoracic vertebra. A small percentage of people are born with a small rib extending on each side from the seventh cervical vertebra. That bone is referred to as a "cervical rib". It is not a true rib. In fact, cervical ribs can cause serious problems by compressing the arterial blood supply at the junction of the neck and the chest. Each true rib bas a groove in its inferior, (lower) edge in which pass an artery, a vein and a nerve to provide for that rib's needs. They also provide the sensory and motor nerve supply, and the circulation to the muscles and the skin along the distribution of each rib.

Beginning at the level of the first thoracic vertebra there are twelve pairs of ribs, each pair articulating in back with a vertebral body. The ribs follow a path that sweeps laterally and downward in back, then turns, going forward, then upward and medially in front. The first through the tenth ribs articulate with the sternum (see below), and with each other through cartilage strips, called the costochondral cartilages. The eleventh and twelfth ribs are called "the floating ribs" because they do not articulate with the sternum, but connect with each other via a cartilaginous articulation.

The sternum, commonly called "the breast bone" is a long narrow shield-shaped bone that extends from the base of the neck to the bottom of the chest. At the bottom of the sternum is a separate small bony structure called the xiphoid process that protrudes forward in many people and can be easily felt. Many of my patients have come to my office fearing that they have felt a tumor in the upper abdomen. What they actually had discovered was the tip of the xiphoid process. The points of attachment of the ribs with the sternum are the costochondral cartilages that allow some flexibility for each rib to move with each breath.

At the uppermost end of the sternum is a thickened, widened area of bone that is called the manubrium. It is at that point that the clavicle, (collarbone) articulates anteriorly to form an important part of the shoulder girdle.

The Shoulder Girdle

The clavicle, commonly called "the collarbone", is a curved bone; roughly J-shaped that extends from its articulation anteriorly with the manubrium of sternum, a joint that is easily felt with the finger, laterally and upward across the top of the chest to join another bone called the scapula.

The scapula commonly called "the wing bone" is a large triangular flat bone shaped quite like a bird's wing. It is a long triangle, pointing downward across the upper back. The scapula is actually held n place by strong muscles, extending medially to the spinous processes of the dorsal vertebrae, and laterally and superiorly to the humerus bone of the upper arm. Those muscular attachments enable the scapula to have fairly wide range of motion.

At its upper, forward, outer point, (superior, antero-lateral point) the scapula has two curved, thick, strong bony projections called the acromial process and the coracoid process respectively. The acromial process is where the clavicle joins the scapula. That is the acromioclavicular or A-C joint. Those three components, two from the scapula, and one from the clavicle form the socket for the shoulder joint

The Shoulder Girdle and Upper Arm

The shoulder girdle is a complex structure of bone, tendons, and ligaments that forms the connection of the upper arm to the structures of the chest. The uppermost bone, (most proximal bone) of the arm is the humerus. It is a long, strong cortical bone that has a ball-shaped head that fits into the socket of the shoulder joint, and ends in two knobs, (condyles), that articulate with the bones of the distal arm. The coracoid process of the scapula is part of the shoulder joint where strong muscles and tendons of the arm attach to the shoulder girdle. The acromial and coracoid processes of the scapula and the ball-shaped head of the humerus with their respective muscles, tendons and ligaments form the shoulder joint.

The shoulder joint is the most versatile joint in the body in its capability of wide range of motion. Try it, and compare with any other joint.

The Elbow Joint

This joint is formed by the union of the condyles of the distal end of the humerus and the proximal ends of the two bones of the forearm, the radius and the ulna. Those are long cortical bones of different shapes. The radius is a thick, strong bone hat extends on the lateral, (thumb) side of the forearm from elbow to the wrist joint. The ulna is a much thinner bone on the medial side of the forearm, also extending from elbow to wrist. They unite with the humerus in a way that allows limited range of motion, but excellent stability. Their range of motion combined with that of the humerus gives the upper extremity a wonderful range of motion. The proximal end of the ulna is a curved projection, called the olecranon process that stabilizes the elbow very well in its articulation with the humerus.

The Wrist Joint And The Hand

The distal ends of the radius and the ulna articulate with eight small carpal bones to form the wrist joint. The names and detailed description of the carpal bones are important to an orthopedist, or a hand surgeon, but would only be excessively detailed for this text. The anatomy and spatial arrangement of those eight small bones is miraculous in that they articulate comfortably with the two large bones of the forearm while providing a base for independent motion of the five metacarpal bones of the hand.

The metacarpal bones are clearly visible and palpable in most hands. They are long, slender cortical bones that extend from the carpal bones of the wrist to the phalangeal bones of the fingers. Those joints are called the metacarpo-phalangeal joints, or M-P joints. The M-P joints provide a solid based for the motion of the fingers.

It is worth noting that the tendons that operate the metacarpal bones and the fingers originate in the muscles of the forearm and pass, together with motor and sensory nerves through a series of compartments called the carpal tunnels. Those tunnels are lined with lubricating synovial membranes. The tendons attach to the bones of the hands and the fingers. Overwork fatigue of those tendons causes swelling of the tendons. The swelling exerts pressure on the nerves within the tunnels. That is the cause of "carpal tunnel syndrome" that has become so prevalent since the advent of the age of computers.

The finger bones, called the phalanges, are operated by a combination of muscles from the forearm and muscles that originate on the finger bones, extending from finger-to finger. The thumb, referred to as "the first finger" has two bones, the proximal and distal phalanges, and articulates with the first metacarpal bone. The other four fingers have three bones each, referred to as the proximal, middle and distal phalanges. They each articulate with the metacarpal bone of the same number, from two to five.

This completes our anatomical tour of the bony structures of the chest, shoulders and upper extremities. Now we will turn our attention to the bony anatomy of the pelvis and lower extremities.

The Pelvis

In the anatomical tour of the vertebral column we saw that the lumbar spine ended in an articulation between the fifth lumbar vertebra and a bone called the sacrum. Articulating with the sacrum on either side is a large curved cancellous bone called the ilium, forming the famous sacro-iliac joints that are blamed for being the site of so many complaints of low back pain. In reality it would be very rare to have low back pain as the result of any significant injury to the sacro-iliac joint. Those joints have broad surfaces that are tightly held together by strong ligaments, and have virtually no mobility. In the vast majority of cases such pain is probably related to musculo-ligamentous injury in that area, or to a more serious problem involving the spinal nerves and intervertebral space in the painful area.

The Hip Joint

The ilium curves anteriorly to form a strong joint on either side with two other pelvic bones called the ischium and the pubis. Together the sacrum, ilium, ischium and pubic bones form the bones of the pelvic girdle. In the lateral aspects of the pelvis where the ilium, ischium and pubis meet, a bony depression or cup is formed. That depression, called the acetabulum, is the cup into which the head of the femur fits to form the hip joint.

The Bones Of The Leg

The femur, which is the thighbone, is the longest and strongest bone in the body. It is formed of dense cortical bone. At its upper, (proximal) end the femur is curved to an angle of approximately forty five degrees for a distance of four to six inches, depending on the size of the individual. The superior end is a smoothly rounded ball that fits into the acetabulum to form a ball and socket joint. The ball shaped portion is called the head of the femur. The segment that travels at an angle to the rest of the femur is called the neck of the femur, and the long portion is called the shaft of the femur. The hip joint has a very good range of motion in all directions, although it is far less than the range of motion of the shoulder joint.

At its lower or distal end the femur ends in two large rounded knobs that are called the medial and lateral condyles of the femur. Those condyles articulate with the bones of the lower leg, the tibia and the fibula, forming the knee joint.

The tibia is a broad, strong bone located on the medial side of the leg. It has two cup-shaped depressions that connect with the condyles of the femur, supporting the weight borne by the femur. The fibula, located laterally to the tibia is a long, slender bone that is connected to the tibia by strong ligaments.

Although this book has purposely omitted a detailed description of the muscular anatomy of the extremities (because of its complexity), it is necessary at this point to comment on the two largest muscle groups in the thigh. The long muscles on the posterior aspect of the thigh are called the hamstring muscles. They provide the major power for flexion of the knee joint. On the anterior surface of the thigh are the quadriceps muscles that are principally responsible for the extension of the knee joint.

The quadriceps muscles end in a strong tendon that goes across the knee joint, inserting on the upper anterior surface of the tibia of the lower leg.

Embedded and supported within the quadriceps tendon is a triangular, but rounded bone called the patella. The common name for the patella is "the kneecap". The patella protects and stabilizes the knee joint.

The Bones Of The Ankle And The Foot

The tibia and fibula of the leg extend to form the ankle joint where they articulate with the talus, which is the first large bone of the foot, to form the ankle joint. It is a hinge-type of joint, held together by very strong ligaments.

The foot is divided into three bony sections, similarly to the bones of the hand and wrist. The proximal bones are the tarsus, which articulates with another large bone, the calcaneus (the heel bone), the middle bones: the metatarsals, and the distal-most bones the phalanges. The tarsal bones articulate with the tibia and fibula proximally, forming the heel. Distally they articulate with the five metatarsal bones. Each of the metatarsal bones articulates at its distal end with a toe. The bones of the toes are similar to those of the hand in that the first toe, (big toe, or great toe) has two bones and all the others have three bones. As in the hand, the bones of the toes are called "phalanges", proximal and distal on the first toe, and proximal, middle, and distal on the other four.

The muscle control of the foot comes mainly from the leg with auxiliary control from muscles extending from bone-to bone within the foot.

Our anatomic tour of the skeletal system has reached its conclusion. Now we will look at the disorders of bones.

COMMON DISORDERS OF BONE

Traumatic Fractures

The most common disorder of bone is fracture, which means in its simplest form, a broken bone. Traumatic fractures, due to injury, are usually straightforward and easily understood. There are "displaced fractures", in which the bone is completely broken and the broken ends separated, and "incomplete fractures", in which the break does not extend completely through the bone. Another classification is "simple fracture", in which the bone is broken, but does not protrude through the skin, and "compound fracture" in which a broken bone end has pierced the skin. There are fractures in which the bone is shattered into multiple fragments. Those are called "comminuted fractures".

In most cases compound fracture are more serious than simple fractures because of the danger of infection in the wound, and possibly in the fractured bone.

In practical terms "simple fractures" can be extremely complicated and difficult to repair, depending upon the nature and location of the fracture.

Pathologic Fractures

Pathologic fractures are more complex because they are due to some underlying disease process. The most common underlying problem is osteoporosis, a metabolic problem in which the bones become deficient in calcium and become soft and lose their strength. When a bone is osteoporotic it can break due to a minor trauma or with no memorable trauma at all. Osteoporosis will be discussed in the next section.

Fractures due to osteoporosis make us "grow shorter" with age. The cause is softening of the bone of the thoracic and lumbar vertebrae. Because there are seventeen bones in the combined thoracic and lumbar regions, a small degree of compression can add up to a substantial loss of height. In most cases that is a painless process because the compression of the vertebrae occurs very gradually. Osteoporosis is also a common cause of fracture of the hip in the elderly. The most frequent fractures of the hip occur in the portion called the femoral neck following a minor fall while walking or standing. Quite often only after the fracture occurs is the osteoporosis of the hip first diagnosed.

Another example of combined pathologic and traumatic fracture is that in which a person who has osteoporosis falls in a sitting position. One or more vertebrae can compress as a result of the fall. Because of the sudden compression due to the fall there is great pain which can persist for a long time. That is a very common cause of vertebral fracture.

A more complicated cause of pathologic fracture is that due to cancer of the bone. Quite commonly the cancer progresses slowly and is asymptomatic until the fracture occurs in the weakened bone. X-Rays then reveal the presence of the cancer. The treatment of such a fracture requires attention to the underlying cancer as well as the orthopedic care.

Dislocations

In its simplest form dislocation is the name given to an injury in which the bones that form a joint are removed from their normal positions. These injuries occur chiefly in the bones of the extremities. The maneuver to return a dislocated bone to its proper location is called "reduction" of the dislocated bone.

Traumatic dislocation of the shoulder is extremely common. It occurs when the humerus is somehow forced from its position within the socket of the shoulder joint. The head of the humerus can be dislocated either anteriorly or posteriorly from its normal position. The dislocation is painful, but in most cases can be reduced by traction distally while rotating the humerus back into its normal position. Dislocations of fingers and toes are commonly seen and usually reduced without difficulty. Dislocations of the elbow are seen much less frequently.

There can be serious complications if in the course of the dislocation there is damage to muscles, ligaments, tendons, nerves or blood vessels in the region of the joint. Another complication that occurs quite frequently is that in the trauma of the dislocation there was serious damage to the soft tissues of the joint capsule. That usually requires some type of surgical procedure to mend the tear, or rupture of the damaged component to prevent future dislocation

Another condition that causes dislocations is congenital malformation of a joint. That is a common cause of dislocation of the hip joint. If, in the course of embryonic development an individual has been given a very shallow acetabulum in one or both hip joints the hip can dislocate easily and frequently. That condition should be discovered early in infancy and reconstructive surgery should be done as early as possible.

Congenital Disorders of Bone

Congenital deformities are unfortunately quite common. They include extra or missing fingers or toes and other misshapen or absent bones. One very common example is the congenitally shallow acetabulum, as discussed above. Whenever possible, surgical correction should be done as early as possible.

Spina bifida is one of the most serious of congenital deformities. It is due to faulty embryonic development of the vertebral column in which there is incomplete closure of the bony structure of the spine. That results in some degree of defect in the protective tube that encloses the spinal cord. Spina bifida can vary from minimal deformity of the vertebral column causing little or no symptOms to very extensive deformity that can lead to permanent neurologic dysfunction or to premature death.

Infections of Bone

Osteomyelitis is the name given to infection of bone. The infecting organism is most often bacterial. Osteomyelitis is frequently the result of an injury that directly involves bone, but it can also occur as the result of the deposition in a bone of bacteria from a blood-borne infection from some remote site.

In most cases the treatment of osteomyelitis is long and difficult because of the very restricted nature of the blood supply via the small canaliculi within the bones. Frequently the treatment requires the daily intravenous administration of antibiotics over a prolonged period of time. In some cases surgical removal of the infected portion of the bone is necessary.

Metabolic Disorders of Bone

The one disorder that is most familiar is the condition called rickets that occurs as the result of deficiency of vitamin D in the diet, particularly in the early formative years of childhood. The result of that deficiency is the inability to retain calcium in the bones. The bones are soft, causing marked bowing of the legs among other bony problems. Ensuring a good supply of calcium and vitamin D in the child's diet can prevent this condition.

Parathyroid abnormalities and pituitary tumors can also cause severe bony disorders, as can chronic diseases of the digestive and urinary systems that cause wasting of protein and minerals from the body.

Osteoporosis is the chief form of metabolic bone disorder. In the post-menopausal years osteoporosis is common in women who do not take a hormonal supplement or some other type of medication that enables the body to retain calcium to be deposited in the matrix of the bones. Osteoporosis is most common in blonde, blue-eyed women and least common in women of African heritage.

Osteoporosis is also quite common in elderly men, usually associated with the hormonal changes of aging.

Cancer of Bone

In most cases cancer involving bone is the result of blood-borne metastasis of cancer cells from cancer in an organ elsewhere in the body. In men it is quite common for cancer of the prostate to metastasize to bone. In women the most likely primary site is cancer of the breast.

It is a very bad sign to have bony metastasis because it is a certainty that the cancer has escaped its primary site and has sent cells out into the body. The likelihood of other metastases being present is quite high in most cases. Lung and brain are also favorite sites for metastases from prostate and breast.

Primary cancer of bone is far less common than the metastatic variety. It is usually found because of pin or fracture in the site of the cancer. The treatment is usually very difficult, sometimes involving a combination of radiation and chemotherapy, and in some cases, surgical removal of the affected bone.

THE JOINTS—ANATOMY AND PHYSIOLOGY

There are three kinds of joints; those that move, those that are fixed, and those that have limited mobility. Examples of fixed joints are the bone-to-bone connections of the pelvic bones. They have strong ligamentous connections but do not flex. Joints with limited mobility are typified by those involving the ribs. There are cartilaginous connections between the ribs and the thoracic vertebrae, and the ribs and the sternum, allowing a limited range of motion with inspiration and expiration.

We will limit our discussion in this section to those joints that move.

All moveable joints have virtually the same anatomy, ranging from the large joints of the hips, knees and shoulders to those of the fingers and toes.

Describing the joints from inside out, one may think of the simple, basic concept of bone-to-bone connection. However, that does not exist. Covering the articulating ends of each bone is a layer of thick, smooth cartilage that acts as a cushion and a frictionless bearing surface. Next there is a membrane called the synovium that covers the entire inside of the joint. The synovium is a smooth sheet of tissue that contains glands that produce a fluid called synovial fluid. That fluid lubricates the joint and also moistens the joint cartilage. Next there is a sheet of strong fibrous tissue called the joint capsule that lends strength to the joint. Finally are the ligaments, strong material that give the joint its ultimate strength and allows for the range of motion of each joint.

Just outside of the joints are the attachments of the tendons of the muscles that cause the bones to move.

COMMON DISORDERS OF THE JOINTS

Joint Injuries

Joint injuries, occurring as a result of twisting, turning or of overstretching a joint are usually called strains or sprains. The distinction between those terms is very vague. That type of injury most commonly occurs in the wrist, the ankle and the knee. The symptoms and signs are sudden severe pain and swelling of the joint, usually intensely aggravated by motion or bearing weight. The swelling is caused by an outpouring of fluid from the synovium of the injured joint. That is the body's way of protecting the injured joint. It is analogous to the outpouring of fluid to form a blister in the process of inflammation. The pain is caused by stretching of the joint capsule by the outpouring of fluid, stimulating the local pain receptors. In severe sprains there is bleeding into the affected joint caused by the breaking of local small blood vessels. Such joints often become warm to touch.

In injuries involving ankles or wrists, where small bones are involved there is always the danger of fracture. For that reason it is always best to have the joint examined by a physician, and probably to have X-Rays taken.

In cases in which the joint swelling is extreme because of the outpouring of synovial fluid the joint capsule is stretched causing severe pain. In those cases it is common for the physician to withdraw fluid from the joint space with a needle. That usually relieves the pain considerably.

Penetrating injuries of any joint, such as those caused by a nail, thorn, or any sharp object should be taken very seriously because of the possibility of implanting an infection that might lead to serious damage to the joint surfaces. Those injuries should be treated professionally very promptly.

In an injury in which there is twisting or sharp bending while running or walking, as in a football player being tackled hard, or struck hard enough to fall, there is always the danger of damage to the ligamentous structures of the joint. This is particularly true of knee injuries. A careful evaluation of the joint by a trained person is essential to diagnose such damage promptly.

INFLAMMATORY DISEASES OF THE JOINTS

Most of the joints of the body can become involved in most kinds of inflammatory diseases. True to our definition of inflammation, an inflammatory disease of joints is called "arthritis". The most common forms of arthritis are osteoarthritis and rheumatoid arthritis. The arthritis of psoriasis and of gout is also quite common.

In addition to the inflammation of joints there are common injuries of structures related to the joints. Typical of those are bursitis and tendinitis. A bursa, in Latin, is a pocket. There are structures related to the knee, the elbow, and the shoulder that facilitate the motion of those joints that are called "pre-patellar", "olecranon", and "sub-deltoid" bursae respectively. An injury to any of those , referred to as "bursitis" can cause pain, limitation of motion, and local heat and swelling. Bursitis is a common injury and can usually be treated by any physician familiar with that condition, with good results. Tendinitis, as it sounds, means inflammation of a tendon, usually as the result of injury. That injury can also usually be treated with good results by any trained physician.

Osteoarthritis

Osteoarthritis is the most common arthritic disease. It usually occurs in people past their mid-forties. It can involve any of the Joints, but is most frequently seen in the hips, knees, wrists, hands and feet. Traditionally, osteoarthritis has been classed as a disease of "wear and tear", due to long hard use of the joints. More recent thinking has classed this disease as an inflammatory disorder, in the auto-immune family of diseases.

The cause is unknown. The distinguishing symptoms and signs are pain and stiffness of the affected joints. Swelling and pain of the knees and of the distal and proximal interphalangeal joints of the fingers and toes, but not the metacarpo-or metatarso-phalangeal joints, (as they are affected in the case of rheumatoid arthritis). There can be severe outpouring of synovial fluid with swelling of the involved joint capsules. The synovium becomes greatly swollen and the disease process ultimately destroys the articular cartilage of the joint. Osteoarthritis is an extremely common and destructive disease of the elderly.

The current treatment of early osteoarthritis at this state of the art involves the use of non-steroidal anti-inflammatory drugs, (NSAIDS), by mouth, and non-stressing exercises to maintain joint mobility. In some joints, especially the knees, there is an outpouring of synovial fluid into the affected joints. That is commonly treated by the aspiration (removal by needle) of the fluid and the injection of a corticosteroid medication into the joint space to reduce the inflammation.

If the disease progresses to the stage of destruction of the articular cartilage some sort of surgical remedy is indicated. In the case of finger joint destruction the insertion of small strips of Teflon, or a similar synthetic material as an artificial joint bearing surface can restore mobility of the joints. Knee joints, probably the most common site of the initial severe manifestations of osteoarthritis, often have severe deterioration of the articular cartilage. It is very common to have arthroscopic surgery done as an initial surgical procedure. That surgery, performed through small incisions with the insertion of a very small video camera enables the surgeon to examine the inside of the joint and to remove particles of broken-up cartilage. That procedure usually gives considerable relief of the joint pain. If the knee joints or the hip joints lose their articular cartilage completely joint replacement surgery is commonly done, usually with good success and the restoration of joint mobility.

Rheumatoid Arthritis

Rheumatoid arthritis is the classical manifestation of an auto-immune disease. It can occur at any age and in either sex. The age at the time of the first onset is quite commonly from the teen years to the fifties or sixties. The first attack of rheumatoid arthritis often follows an episode of streptococcal sore throat. That fact has led to the theory that there is a hyper-immune allergic relationship to prior streptococcal bacterial infections as the precipitating cause.

Rheumatoid arthritis is most often insidious in its progression. In most cases the disease is manifested by pain and tenderness in the involved joints, becoming progressively more severe. The first episode of rheumatoid arthritis can also be explosive in onset, frequently involving multiple movable joints in its first manifestation. It is not uncommon for the initial attack to cause permanent crippling of multiple joints.

Any of the moveable joints in the body can be involved. The joints most commonly involved initially are those of the hands and feet, including the proximal interphalangeal and metacarpo-phalangeal joints in the hands, and the proximal interphalangeal and metatarsophalangeal joints in the feet. The wrists, elbows, shoulders, and the ankles, knees and hip joints are also frequently involved. The synovium becomes inflamed and thickened. The cartilage of the joints is frequently attacked, causing severe damage. As a result the joints can become fused, and unable to move.

This is a devastating disease, requiring very intensive care as soon as possible after the first onset of symptoms. The treatment usually involves the use of corticosteroid medication and NSAIDS. Powerful immunosuppressive medications are frequently used. Although bed rest is often required, some effort to maintain joint mobility is usually made.

After the active disease process subsides the patient usually retains an immunologic problem and there is a tendency for the attacks of inflammation to recur.

Surgical remedies of the residual joint deformities are often deferred because of that tendency. Long-term therapy with some type of immunosuppressive medication is usually required.

Psoriatic Arthritis

Psoriatic arthritis is another auto-immune disease, quite similar to rheumatoid arthritis, but not as explosive, and usually not as severe. The joint manifestations are accompanied by a severe form of inflammatory dermatitis called psoriasis. That disease was discussed in the previous chapter on the skin.

The joint involvement in Psoriatic Arthritis usually includes the distal interphalangeal joints in the hands and feet. There can be a wide range of joints in an asymmetric pattern involved. The joints of the spine are frequently involved, causing permanent stiffness and deformity of the back.

This disease also requires intensive treatment with corticosteroids, NSAIDS, and immuno-suppressive drugs. Permanent deformities, especially of the spine are not unusual.

Gouty Arthritis

Gouty arthritis is the joint manifestation of a metabolic disorder called gout.

The cause of that disease is a congenital deficiency of an enzyme called uricase. That enzyme is responsible for the breakdown of a compound called uric acid, which is one of the products of the metabolism of the protein called Purine. Because of the absence of uricase the uric acid cannot be broken down into its ultimate waste products, ammonia and water, which are normally excreted via the kidneys. Uric acid accumulates in the plasma of the blood, forming crystals. Those crystals can precipitate out of the plasma, lodging in joints and also in the kidneys, forming kidney stones.

The joints most commonly involved are the metatarsophalangeal joints of the big toe, (first toe) on either foot. The result is severe swelling, redness and pain in that joint. Other joints can be involved, but less commonly, and with less severity and visibility.

Gouty arthritis of the big toe is easily seen. The affected joint swells, reddens, and becomes intensely warm, tender and painful. If needle aspiration of that joint is performed the fluid obtained reveals the presence of microscopic crystals of uric acid. There are good medications to treat the joint symptoms of gout, and to minimize the formation of uric acid crystals in the blood.

In most cases the disease is easily managed in the hands of most physicians. Your primary care physician should be contacted at the first sign of symptoms. In most cases there is no necessity for specialist consultation unless complications arise.

Ankylosing Spondylitis (Marie-Stumpell Disease)

This is a joint disorder that chiefly involves the spine. Other joints can be involved, but the main target is the spine.

The cause of the disease is unknown. It affects men approximately three times as often as women. The onset is usually in the second of third decades. The tendency is for the disease to progress throughout the lifetime of the patient.

The first manifestation of this disease is often in the low back and in the sacro-iliac joints of the pelvis. As the disease extends in a cephalad (upward) direction the cartilages between the vertebrae become eroded, causing fusion of the intervertebral joints. That results in a forward- leaning posture that is rigid.

There is no effective treatment of Ankylosing Spondylitis. It is important for the patient to follow a conscientious program of exercise to minimize the deformity. Treatment with NSAIDS and other immunosuppressive drugs has a place early in the course of the disease, but exercise and the use of non-habituating analgesic medications is the best treatment in the long run.

Chapter Eleven
THE BLOOD

OVERVIEW

There are five to six liters of blood in the body of the average male. Females average four to five liters, with variations depending on the size of the individual. Blood has two chief components: the blood cells, and the fluid in which the cells are suspended. There are many classes and types of blood cells, each different in appearance, and having widely different functions and diseases.

The fluids of the blood have multiple compositions, each fluid performing a differing function. Blood serves as a transport medium, carrying nutrients, metabolites and waste products from one part of the body to other parts. Blood is even important as a regulator of body temperature. We will begin our tour with a discussion of the fluids of the blood.

THE FLUIDS OF THE BLOOD

The blood cells are suspended in a fluid called the plasma. Plasma is composed mainly of water in which are suspended or dissolved minerals, carbohydrates, fats and proteins. The plasma acts as a transport vehicle for compounds that are produced by the various organs of the body, such as hormones, and metabolites that are formed by the liver. It has the job of transporting nutrients to all organs and waste products to the kidneys to be excreted from the body.

The protein fraction within the plasma is called the blood serum. Those proteins include metabolites, antibodies, hormones, and other substances that are manufactured by organs of the body, and are being transported to other organs for further metabolism.

BLOOD CLOTTING

Fibrinogen is a protein compound that circulates within the plasma continuously. If a blood vessel anywhere in the body is injured that injured vessel releases a compound called thromboplastin. The presence of that compound triggers a reaction in the blood that causes the fibrinogen that has been held in suspension to become long solid strands of fibrin that form a network to fill the gap in the injured blood vessel. The fibrin network then entraps blood platelets, (see next section) that form a blood clot (thrombus) to stop the bleeding.

The process of thrombus formation is actually more complicated, involving a cascade of events within the blood vessels in which substances called clotting factors come into play in a sequential manner, activating the thromboplastin to become thrombin. Those factors are held in balance by multiple enzymes, also circulating in the blood, that prevent the accidental formation of blood clots. Blood clot formation is an extremely complex process, held in a delicate balance. Diseases of blood clotting, such as hemophilia, are due to the absence or inactivity of those factors.

As wonderful as the process of blood clotting is, it has a serious downside. The events of a coronary heart attack or a stroke are closely involved with the formation of thrombus in the injured blood vessel. That thrombus, if it extends to adjacent vessels greatly increases the damage to the heart or brain by further depriving that organ of blood supply.

Modern emergency treatment of coronary heart attack or stroke is aimed at preventing the extension of the thrombus and whenever possible dissolving the original thrombus

ANTIBODIES

Antibodies, components of the serum proteins, are an important part of the immune system. They are protein molecules that are produced by the liver and spleen in response to the presence of various foreign proteins that are called antigens that threaten the body. Once produced, antibodies circulate in the serum continuously. If the antigen that caused their production is again encountered the antibodies attack the antigen, rendering it harmless to the body. A good example of that is the vaccination process in which a vaccine prepared from inactivated organisms, such as the virus that causes measles is injected into the body. Antibodies against that virus are produced and remain in the blood permanently to protect against succumbing to the live, infective form of the measles virus. Some immunizations must be repeated at intervals in order to maintain the immunity.

THE BLOOD CELLS

The Red Blood Cells

Their name in "doctor-speak" is "erythrocytes". "Erythro" is Greek for red, "cyte" is Greek for cell. They are very small. There are about five million erythrocytes in every milliliter of blood. There are a thousand milliliters in one liter. Since all of us have from four to six liters of blood in circulation there are TRILLIONS of erythrocytes in each of our bodies. The reason they are called "red blood cells" is that they contain an organic compound called hemoglobin that is very rich in iron. Because of hemoglobin the erythrocytes have the capability of taking in oxygen and carbon dioxide. Blood flowing in the arteries, loaded with oxygen is very red. In the veins the blood, poor in oxygen and rich in carbon dioxide has a bluish color.

For an explanation of the mechanism of gas exchange in the blood, and the role of the red blood cells in the handling of oxygen and carbon dioxide see Chapter One, The Respiratory System.

Erythrocytes are made in the marrow of bones. They originate as immature cells, and as the cells become mature they are released into the circulation. In disease states immature cells are sometimes released into the circulation.

The White Blood Cells

The "doctor-speak" name for white blood cells is "leukocytes", derived from the Greek "leuko", meaning white. They are much larger than erythrocytes. There are five to twelve thousand leukocytes in each milliliter of blood, as compared to four to six million per milliliter for erythrocytes.

Leukocytes are divided by their origins, descriptions, and functions into two classes; the agranulocytes and the granulocytes. There are two chief types of agranulocytes. They are called lymphocytes and monocytes. Lymphocytes are chiefly important in the defense against viral infections, such as HIV infection. This is especially true of the T- lymphocytes. The B-lymphocytes are the bearers of antibodies to combat infections of all types. Monocytes have the role of phagocytosis. That expression means that they engulf invading organisms and destroy them.

Granulocytes are very important in protecting the body, chiefly from bacterial infections. When viewed microscopically they have nuclei of various shapes and are therefore called polymorphonuclear leukocytes (many-shaped nucleated white cells). They are commonly called

"polys." There are two different kinds of polys that have different chemical compositions that enable them to be identified when a drop of blood is smeared onto a microscope slide, by using special staining techniques. They are in that way divided into three classes, called neutrophiles, basophiles and eosinophiles. If a severe acute bacterial infection occurs, such as acute appendicitis, there is a great outpouring of neutrophiles and basophiles. They can engulf and destroy invading organisms. In medical lingo a "high white cell count" in the case of an infection means that it is a severe infection and that the body is mounting a strong resistance by producing many polymorphonuclear leukocytes. Eosiniphiles are seen in increased numbers when some type of allergic or immunologic event is in progress or in certain parasitic infestations.

DISORDERS OF THE RED BLOOD CELLS

Anemia

The most commonly seen disorder of the blood is anemia. The term literally means "without blood cells", or "no blood cells". Of course the true meaning, commonly used is "low red blood cell count".

Anemia can be due to a number of widely different causes that are classified as "the anemias". One very common type is that due to severe dietary deficiency, chiefly due to a diet low in iron and/or protein. Probably the most common cause of anemia is chronic loss of blood from the body. That is quite common in women who have heavy menstrual periods and do not compensate for the blood loss with their diet or supplemental iron. Another kind of chronic blood loss is that due to slow bleeding from a gastrointestinal disorder, such as an ulcer or a tumor.

Another kind of anemia is called hemolytic anemia, which is due to some type of disorder that causes red blood cells to break up within the body. Those are congenitally acquired anemias, chiefly sickle cell disease or Mediterranean anemia.

There is anemia due to chronic exposure to toxic substances that depresses the bone marrow, such as that due to lead poisoning. There are anemias due to chronic parasite infestation, such as tapeworm infestation which actually causes chronic blood loss. Finally, there is anemia due to leukemia, a cancer of the white blood cells that overwhelms the blood-forming capability of the bone marrow.

All of those causes of anemia can be diagnosed and treated.

Polycythemia

Polycythemia, a word formed from the Greek "poly", meaning many, "cyte", meaning cell, and "heme", meaning blood, is the name given to the disease, caused by a malignant change in the bone marrow resulting in a great overproduction of red blood cells. The cells are not truly effective as erythrocytes because of defects caused by their very rapid formation. Patients with this disease are in serious danger of obstruction of small blood vessels caused by very great numbers of red blood cells blocking the small vessels. They are also prone to congestive heart failure caused by overload of the capillaries within the lungs.

This disease is relatively easy to diagnose and, in most cases, to treat, but is not curable, requiring lifetime observation and treatment.

DISORDERS OF THE WHITE BLOOD CELLS

Leukemia

This name means "white blood". It is derived from the Greek words meaning white, and blood. The disease is really cancer of the white blood cells. There are two main types of leukemia; acute and chronic. Both are manifested by a significant increase in the number of white blood cells. In acute leukemia the cells involved are chiefly granulocytes, produced in the bone marrow. Chronic leukemia most often involves the agranulocytes that are manufactured in the spleen and lymph nodes. They are really two different diseases. Acute leukemia can occur at any age, but is most often seen in children and young adults. It is a very aggressive disease, causing severe weakness, weight loss and anemia. The anemia occurs because the white blood cells that are being produced are made within the bone marrow, which is where the red blood cells are made. The rampant production of white cells crowds out the red cells, seriously reducing their production. The abnormal white blood cells invade important organs. Diseased white blood cells lack the ability to fight infection, normally the role of healthy granulocytes. Because of this the patient becomes susceptible to infections that would normally not occur in a healthy individual. Infection is commonly the cause of death in acute leukemia. Most acute leukemias are rapidly fatal. Much medical research is currently devoted to the cause and treatment of that terrible disease.

Chronic leukemia is, in most cases, a very different disease. It most often occurs in people over the age of fifty. The cells involved are most often lymphocytes, the white blood cells that are formed in the spleen and lymph nodes, although the monocytes are occasionally involved. Chronic Lymphocytic Leukemia, (CLL) is usually a quite benign disease, as is chronic monocytyic leukemia. Chronic leukemia is most often discovered in the course of a routine blood count when a significant increase in the number of lymphocytes or monocytes is found. These diseases rarely cause serious damage to any organ and do not cause anemia, and usually do not shorten the life of the patient. These leukemias can, in rare cases, transform into acute leukemias which have a poorer prognosis.

Lymphomas

Lymphomas are cancers of the organs that make lymphocytes. The suffix "oma" is used to denote any type of tumor, and so was given to this disease. There are, in general, two kinds of lymphomas: Hodgkin's (named after the doctor who first identified the disease) and non-Hodgkin's lymphoma.

Hodgkin's lymphoma is most often discovered in the course of a routine physical examination in which the doctor finds an enlarged lymph node, liver, or spleen. The disease is also quite often discovered by the patient who feels a lump in the neck, armpit or groin during a shower. This discovery usually leads to a medical workup and surgical removal, (biopsy) of a lymph node or nodes, in order to establish the diagnosis of the disease.

Non-Hodgkin's lymphoma is usually not found that way. It is in most cases an aggressive disease, causing fatigue and malaise, possibly with weight loss that brings the patient to the doctor. A physical examination usually reveals enlargement of multiple lymph nodes, the spleen and the liver. That, again, leads to the medical workup and a surgical biopsy of lymph nodes to establish the diagnosis.

The usual workup for lymphoma involves blood counts, X-Rays, and MRI examination to look for involvement of internal organs and lymph nodes. If the results are consistent with lymphoma a staging operation is commonly done. Staging is a systematic search to determine the extent of the disease. Most modern treatment of all cancers, including lymphomas, is based on the aggressiveness and the extent of the disease at the time that it is diagnosed.

The treatment of lymphomas usually consists of a combination of radiation and chemotherapy. The results with Hodgkin's lymphoma are usually quite good because that disease tends to be less aggressive. Non-Hodgkin's lymphoma has a generally poor prognosis. The disease is usually fatal after a short course.

Chapter Twelve
THE IMMUNE SYSTEM

OVERVIEW

The medical definition of "immune" according to The Encyclopedia Britannica dictionary is "to be protected from disease". Immunology, according to the same source, is "the science which treats of the phenomena and techniques of the protection from disease". Immunology is an extremely complicated body of knowledge and a science that has been the lifelong work of many research scientists and practitioners. I will try my best to make the essence of this information simple and useful.

There are two basic components to the immune system of the body. First, the innate or non-specific components, present from birth, that do not require any previous exposure to the substance that threatens or offends the body. This consists of natural barriers such as the skin and certain elements of the blood, present at birth, such as the cells called phagocytes, which can engulf and destroy invading organisms.

The second component of the immune system requires specific adaptive or learned immunity. That component consists of cells such as lymphocytes and other components called immunoglobulins which are proteins circulating within the serum of the blood.

The lymphocytes of the immune system are labeled T-lymphocytes, or B-lymphocytes, depending on their origin, (thymus or bone marrow). Those terms are frequently seen in the literature of HIV disease.

The immunoglobulins are capable of recognizing viruses and other foreign proteins within the body and making anti-protein molecules, which are called "antibodies." Antibodies can recognize and destroy or inactivate invaders of the body. They also have the unique ability to replicate themselves, creating circulating antibodies that can remain within the blood stream for long periods, or for a lifetime in some cases. That capability is the reason for the routine immunizations against viral diseases that are a part of most of our childhood medical histories.

DISORDERS OF THE IMMUNE SYSTEM

As in most things in life, there is a downside to the workings of the immune system. In many cases the system "works overtime", presumably in its efforts to protect the body. When that occurs the end product can be the phenomenon called "allergy".

The manifestations of allergy are well known, such as runny nose, wheezing, and skin rashes. The invading substances are called Allergens or Antigens.

The reaction between allergens and antibodies often causes the release of histamine, or histamine-like substances from the involved tissue. That initiates the process of inflammation, which was discussed at the beginning of this book. The treatment most commonly used for allergic reactions is the administration of "anti-histamine" medications, non-steroidal anti-inflammatory drugs (NSAIDS), or corticosteroid preparations commonly called "cortisone drugs" to suppress the inflammation process.

Disorders of the immune system can also be very severe, leading to death or severe permanent disabilities. Let's take a look at the most frequently seen of those severe disorders.

DISEASES AND DISORDERS KNOWN TO BE DUE TO IMMUNE REACTIONS FOLLOWING EXPOSURE TO SPECIFIC ANTIGENIC SUBSTANCES

A list of the most common disorders includes:

Allergic Rhinitis and Sinusitis

Bronchial Asthma (in most cases)

Allergic Dermatitis: Contact allergies (specific allergenic substances)

Penicillin and other drug sensitivities—skin rash and generalized symptoms

Specific food intolerances—gastrointestinal dysfunction

Rheumatic Fever—(a major disease following throat infections due to Type A Streptococcal bacteria in genetically susceptible individuals)

There are many more disorders due to specific exposure to antigenic substances and due to apparent over-reaction of the immune system.

DISEASES AND DISORDERS DUE TO IMMUNE REACTIONS NOT FOLLOWING EXPOSURE TO SPECIFIC ANTIGENIC SUBSTANCES

This is an extremely complex subject, but a very important one. This author will attempt to explain it to the best of his ability without getting lost in the details or omitting the essential important parts.

In the above discussion of the immune system mention was made of the ability of the body to create antibodies, modeling them after known antigens that are purposely introduced into the body. That is the basis of the process of conferring immunity against common virus infections by giving childhood immunization shots.

In addition to the "good" antibodies that we create by giving immunizations there also are "bad" antibodies that can circulate within the blood plasma. Those antibodies can be identified by laboratory tests. The source or means by which they are created is unknown. The result of their action is a body of diseases called

AUTO-IMMUNE DISORDERS

The scientific description of those disorders is "Disorders in which the immune system produces AUTOANTIBODIES to an endogenous antigen with consequent injury to tissues." The mystery word in that definition is endogenous. No one knows why or how such antigens exist or how they work to create those antibodies. It is a common enough phenomenon so that the names of the disease states that it causes will probably be known to most readers, or have been discussed previously in this book. They include:

Hashimoto's thyroiditis (the most common cause of hypothyroidism).

Rheumatoid Arthritis

Grave's Disease (toxic hyperthyroidism)

Subacute Lupus Erythematosus (a severe multi-system disease)

Myasthenia Gravis

Scleroderma

Glomerulonephritis

Temporal Arteritis and other forms of Arteritis

That is a partial list of the disorders that are classed as "Auto-immune" in origin. It is evident that it is a very significant group of diseases and disorders. In most cases abnormal antibodies can be identified. The treatment is very complicated, usually requiring some form of replacement or support of the failed organ or system and the intensive use of corticosteroids and drugs to suppress the inflammatory reaction.

The specialty of Immunology is a combination of Laboratory Science and practical medicine. Most internists and trained Family Physicians have some education in the management of auto-immune diseases and can manage most cases. Consultation with Immunologists is usually available in communities having a medical school or major medical center. Immunologic consultation is very helpful in severe cases of auto-immune disorders.

Chapter Thirteen
THE MIND-BODY CONNECTION

In the chapter on the nervous system quite a lot of time and effort was spent in an attempt to describe the brain and its amazing complexity in a relatively simple form. It's quite likely that the readers and I will agree that the brain is where the process of thinking most likely goes on, but then the question arises; "does the working of that wonderful electro-chemical apparatus qualify as the sum and substance of THE MIND?" Nowhere in my years of experience as a physician and a teacher, or in my reading, have I found a satisfactory answer to that question. At this point I would like to offer my own thoughts on that subject.

The mind is the sum of our thoughts, conscious and unconscious, our true feelings and biases, some of which we are aware, and most of which we are probably unaware, and the product of all of the experiences of our lives.

The conscious part of the mind is the repository of everything we have ever made the effort to learn, and a great deal more that we have learned without trying. Part of that repository of information is lodged in a deeper level of awareness that is referred to in psychiatric terms as the "subconscious" mind. That part of the mind is the source of thinking, orientation and behavior that occur apparently without conscious effort. The ability to recall and use information that might be very old and very obscure or to retain foreign languages that we have not used for a very long time is really amazing, and a lot of that goes on at a subconscious level.

Psychiatric study has shown that the ability of the subconscious mind to retain information and impressions is equally amazing.

Most, but not all of the conscious actions that we perform are initiated by references to conscious memories and purposefully learned material. Some of our behavior, such as becoming hungry and having our mouths water because of delicious cooking smells is not really a conscious effort, but the action of our autonomic nervous system responding to stimuli from our unconscious mind. The same can be said for most sexual responses to stimuli that are initially perceived by the conscious mind, which then relays the information to the subconscious mind which then triggers the autonomic nervous system to initiate sexual arousal.

If everything we do required direction and response from our conscious nervous system our bodies and our lives, and quite likely the history of mankind would be very different than they are.

The most important part of this chapter is the concept of the relationship between the subconscious mind and the body. In the chapter on the nervous system there was considerable discussion of the autonomic nervous system and its function and importance. To re-state briefly, the autonomic nervous system has two parts: the sympathetic and the parasympathetic systems. The sympathetic system prepares our bodies for "fight or flight" reactions.

These enable the body to deal with stressful emergencies and severe sudden challenges such as might have befallen our ancestors when attacked by a saber tooth tiger. Today's person might have to face a domestic crisis or a bad letter from the I.R.S. Our heart races, the blood pressure rises, blood is shunted from the skin and digestive system to the muscles, heart and brain and we prepare to flee or to fight. The parasympathetic part of the autonomic nervous system, in general, has the opposite effect. It causes the heart to slow down, and reverses the other effects of the sympathetic system. In most cases the sympathetic nervous system, functioning on commands from the unconscious part of the brain, is the villain. It over-compensates in the flight-or fight response, causing damage to the body.

This book is really not the place for a complete discussion of these matters but let's try to touch on the most important facts of the mind-body connection.

The proper name for this type of problem is "psycho-somatic disorders". The term "somatic" refers to the entire body. "Psycho", the part played by the brain and the mind. The most important elements in this relationship are the autonomic nervous system, the endocrine glands (mainly the pituitary, adrenals and thyroid) and that part of the brain that is responsible for the storage and retrieval of unconscious memory.

The target organs that are affected by psycho-somatic dysfunction include practically every part of the body. It is generally accepted among experts in psychiatry that the heart, blood vessels, respiratory system (chiefly the bronchial passages in asthma), stomach, small and large intestines male and female reproductive systems, skin, hair, musculoskeletal systems, and probably most of all, the behavior of men, women , and even children can be affected by psycho-somatic dysfunction.

At the risk of seriously over-simplifying the processes of psycho-somatic disorders here s this author's concept of how the system works. Chiefly as the result of activity of the subconscious mind an anxiety state is created. The brain perceives that an ongoing stress situation is present. That causes the sympathetic nervous system to stimulate the target organs to prepare for flight or fight. The pituitary gland produces a lot of TSH hormone that stimulates the thyroid gland to produce and secrete thyroxine hormone that increases the heart rate and the rate of metabolism of many of the body tissues. The sympathetic nerves also stimulate the adrenal medulla to produce and secrete more epinephrine (adrenaline) that also increases the heart rate and the blood pressure, and increases neuro-muscular tone. Gastro-intestinal motility is increased, resulting in frequent loose stools. Gastric acid production is increased, causing irritation of the duodenal mucosa, possibly leading to peptic ulcer formation. Menstrual periods become irregular and can cease altogether. Libido and sexual activity, both male and female, are usually diminished. Muscle tone and tension increases, causing tension headaches and sore muscles. Hives, eczema and other skin rashes can occur. All of the foregoing can occur as the result of over-activity of the sympathetic nervous system in a state of stress-anxiety. The longer the anxiety state persists, the greater the potential damage to the body. Most of the symptoms and signs just described are physical manifestations, distinct clues to the fact that a sustained anxiety-stress state is present. There are usually abnormalities upon laboratory testing. The conclusion is usually reached that the individual would benefit from some sort of treatment or help.

The other side of the coin in psycho-somatic disorders is the situation in which the individual has subjective symptoms that are NOT accompanied by physical findings or any abnormal laboratory tests. That kind of disorder can be very difficult for the physician to diagnose and to manage. The absence of physical signs and laboratory abnormalities gives no clues that would lead to the diagnosis, yet the patient complains of severe, sometimes unbearable and indescribable pain, or other symptoms. In some cases there is real weight loss and wasting of muscle tissue, leading to performing multiple specialized X-Rays and tests to rule out physically-based disease that could and should be treated. In such cases no abnormalities are found upon testing.

Such patients often go from doctor to doctor to attempt to find relief of their symptoms. They quite often have unnecessary and unhelpful treatments, including surgeries. In many such cases psychiatric consultation would be appropriate and probably helpful. Those patients sometimes choose suicide in their despair.

Psycho-somatic disorders are quite common in all sectors of our society. They do not favor the wealthy or the poor. They are responsible for a substantial share of the national health care budget.

Unfortunately, there are medical professionals in every community who recognize and prey upon these unfortunate people, quite often giving treatment that is ineffective, expensive, and sometimes dangerous. Sadly, many people who choose that kind of treatment could be helped by more caring and competent and honest physicians.

Chapter Fourteen
MAINTENANCE

In the course of this handbook we have spent considerable time together looking at the construction, functioning, and the most common disorders of this wonderful and complicated machine, the human body.

Now is the time at which I, the author, am faced with one further requirement that is found in any proper Owner's Manual. That is to write a maintenance program for this wonderful machine. Unfortunately, I do not have the luxury of consulting with the designers and engineers of the machine, as in any automobile owner's handbook. For this task I must rely on my own experience and knowledge of physiology and medicine and that which I have derived from my studying and communicating with my wonderful patients. I have also done my best to research the best current scientific thinking in a variety of medical fields.

My first thought on the subject was to advise the readers to use their own good "common sense" about the maintenance of their bodies. However, after taking a good look at the current status of health and disease in this country I have come to the conclusion that a significant proportion of our diseases are self-inflicted. This has led me to the conclusion that many of us lack "common sense" or have a distorted concept of that attribute. For that reason I will set down my own concept of good maintenance of the body and hope that the readers will find within these words some common sense.

STOP HURTING YOURSELF

Throughout this book are numerous references to the fact that obesity (being seriously overweight) is the main cause of high blood pressure, heart disease, strokes, and diabetes. There is a serious worldwide epidemic of those disorders and the main cause, by far, is the epidemic of obesity. It is most severe in children and in people of African descent, but it involves all ages and races, in "developed" nations. The epidemic is due to overeating, mainly of fats, carbohydrates, and "fast foods" and to under-exercising.

There is no "fast fix" to this terribly serious problem. It requires a real change in lifestyle. There is no official "best reducing diet." The closest that I know of is the Weight Watchers type of diet that includes every kind of food, but in the structure of a reduced quantity, combined with the strict minding of caloric content. If other kinds of diet work best for you then go for it, but be sure you are getting proper nutrition. In most instances some supervision of the diet program is advisable for best results.

Exercise means different things to different people. A major start is the severe rationing of time spent in front of a computer or a TV set or a Game Boy. Walking is available to almost everyone, and to my thinking is the best all-round exercise for most people. Some structure to your walking is necessary. A good way to start is to set a minimum time of thirty minutes of walking at as brisk a pace as possible. As you get better at it and as your condition improves the time and the pace can be increased.

Advanced age and poor health really do not prevent doing some type of exercise. With only rare exceptions there is some kind of exercise for nearly everyone, even if it is done in a chair or flat in bed. Recreational exercise such as bicycling, sports, or swimming is very good. Gym workouts are "icing on the cake" for those who so choose. Whatever the choice, my best advice, to borrow a slogan from Nike TV commercials is: "JUST DO IT."

NO SMOKING ALLOWED

SMOKING is a widely discussed cause of lung cancer, emphysema, many chronic diseases of the lungs, and of heart disease. Smoking is publicly discouraged on TV, billboards, and in the media in general; yet smokers pay a stiff price for their smokes and pay the price of their health for the pleasure. It is not easy, but stopping smoking is the best thing a smoker can do for self, family, and society. There are good medications to make it easier to stop. There is, however, one true fact; no one can quit who does not want to quit. It is really up to you.

ALCOHOL AND OTHER ADDICTING DRUGS

Not much has to be said about the damaging effects of those substances. Alcohol, in moderation, is good for most adults. Some societies raise their children with small amounts of alcohol regularly. The real problem is that of the person who, for whatever reason, has an addictive personality. That person cannot stop in time. The daily limit recommended by A.A. and many health authorities is three beers, three (four ounce) glasses of wine, three ounces of strong alcohol, or any combination of those, totaling no more than three. The addictive person must avoid all alcohol completely.

Narcotics and addictive drugs have taken a terrible toll in human lives in this country and others around the world. The best advice is to avoid any initial contact with them. Once the habit has become established it is worth any effort or treatment to stop. There is competent and caring help available in most communities for those who reach out.

In addition to the first commandment, "stop hurting yourself"; with its list of "don'ts" there is a list of positive ways to provide good maintenance for your body. My common sense list goes something like this.

HELP YOURSELF

If it is at all possible find a doctor with whom you can be comfortable and above all, who will talk to you and LISTEN to you. Regardless of educational credentials, the most important things doctors have to offer their patients are their time, attention and their interest in the patient. If you feel that you are not getting those from your doctor it might be time to find another doctor. Have regular checkups to enable early detection and correction of disorders. Those things are sometimes hard to get in this day of "managed" health care, but it is worth the effort to keep trying.

NUTRITION

Diet choices should include all the food groups with attention to the total caloric content. Fad diets usually fade away. For young and healthy individuals all the vitamins and nutritional supplements that you need can be found at your local market. Meats, fish and seafood in moderation are healthful. Grains, salads, and other vegetables, eggs and dairy foods in most cases have all the nutrition you need. To repeat; my best advice for an effective and sustainable weight loss program is to sign up with Weight Watchers and to be a regular participant.

When we reach "middle age", an elastic tern, the body undergoes changes that are simply due to the aging process. This, I call "paying our dues." Some systems of the body start to require extra nutritional support. At that time it is a good idea to start taking some sort of nutritional supplement on a regular basis. Specific supplements, such as those recommended for macular degeneration of the eyes are quite helpful. Your doctor should be able to advise you of what supplements to take.

Regular exercise is really a "must" for people of all ages, regardless of health status or physical limitations. It is common sense to start slowly, monitor how you feel, and gradually increase your exercise to maximum tolerance. Do not exercise to exhaustion-save something for tomorrow. Some sort of workout every day is really the best for your body, and also very relaxing and helpful for your mind.

FOR SENIORS: EXERCISE YOUR BRAIN

Avoid idleness. Never "kill time." Time is too precious to kill. Keep your mind and your memory working. This is especially important. The maxim, "use it or lose it" is very true. Do crossword puzzles, read books, or listen to books on tape. Play card games or other games requiring memory and intellectual choices.

At all times try to remember to "push back." Senility is not inevitable at any age. If it becomes evident that your "mental muscles" are weakening work hard to strengthen them by some of the exercises suggested above. Good conversation is good mental exercise so talk with people and invite them to talk with you.

These thoughts are my best effort at giving "common sense" general advice. Remember that your doctor is important to you. You should be able to feel free to consult him or her about health issues and to expect a reasonable response. Have regular examinations. Remember that you must be the principal caretaker of your own body and your mind.

www.ingramcontent.com/pod-product-compliance
Lightning Source LLC
Chambersburg PA
CBHW071355170526
45165CB00001B/49
* 9 7 8 1 4 3 9 2 3 1 0 2 9 *